I have no affiliation with any companies or individuals who manufacture, sell or distribute any products recommended in this book.

Table of Contents

Preface

When you're a teenager, pimples or spots are seen as part of growing up, like some sort of rite of passage to adulthood. But for some of us the spots multiply out of control, and keep on coming, not just through college or university, but after graduation and on into our twenties and beyond.

The pimples sometimes become cysts, the cysts heal and leave all kinds of scars with crazy names such as keloid, boxcar and ice pick. We obsess over the state of our skin in the mirror. We try creams from the pharmacy. When they don't work, we go to see doctors and dermatologists who prescribe us stronger creams and all sorts of pills. They may work for a few weeks and we feel elated, finally we can start living again.

But then the acne comes back and our hope is cruelly taken away. For some, that's fine. But for most of us, it's not. We realise that, from being just a minor nuisance in the beginning, acne has slowly taken over our lives.   Without realising it, acne has affected everything we do: our job, the way we communicate, our hobbies, the food we eat, our relationships: everything. The overwhelming feeling is one of hopelessness. "What can I do?" "How can I get my life back?"

This is where this guide can help. I suffered from severe acne for over twenty years. Now, I am acne free.

I'm confident that, if you follow the advice laid out in this guide, you too will be acne free.

I will review everything I tried in over twenty years of fighting acne. What works - very little - and what doesn't work - almost everything. I will also talk about what causes acne and what makes some people more susceptible than others. I will talk about food and lifestyle, and what habits make the problem worse.

Most importantly, I will tell you how to be free of acne and how to stay free of acne.

There is special advice for people of different skin colours and particular advice for women. Also, I will talk about how to deal with scars once you are free of active acne.

Throughout the guide, I will reference peer reviewed scientific research as often as I can - there are no wooly, back of a cigarette packet solutions presented here. What's more, during all this, I promise I will try to talk to you in an honest and non-patronising way. So, let's begin.

1. Why Do You Have Acne?

When it comes to acne, everyone professes to be an expert. "Chocolate gives you spots". "You need to have better personal hygiene". "It's the stress of your job".

Some of the advice may hold an element of truth, but most of it is nonsense. For example, personal hygiene. True, it's important to wash your face and body to remove grease and grime from your skin, but washing too frequently and/or too aggressively will actually cause sebaceous glands to produce more oil and hence more acne. Twice a day is just fine. In my experience, acne sufferers usually take extra care about cleanliness, and have better a personal hygiene regime than most people.

So if poor personal hygiene isn't the reason you have acne, then what is? We know how spots form. Dead skin cells and excess oil (sebum) from sebaceous glands block skin pores. *P.acnes* bacteria, loving the conditions inside the blocked pore, multiply. This leads to inflammation, resulting in pustules (pimples) and sometimes, more seriously, cysts and nodules. The skin on the face, chest, neck and back contains a high density of pores, which is why we are more prone to spots in these areas.

The key points for acne sufferers are why do we produce excess oil in the first place and why are we prone to getting blocked pores? The reason most of us start to get acne during our teens is hormones. The levels of androgen hormones such as testosterone (present in both men and women) increase at puberty and can cause sebaceous glands to produce excess sebum and so acne. However, hormone levels usually stabilise as most people get older, and the number of acne breakouts reduces.

So what about adults? Why do we still get acne, into our twenties, thirties and beyond? The fact is that the medical community isn't 100% sure. Like most drugs, acne medication is targeted at the symptoms, not the root causes of the problem. So doctors and dermatologists prescribe us skin creams to open pores, antibiotics to kill bacteria, and accutane to reduce sebum production. This leaves us at the mercy of people touting "miracle cures" on the internet, which promise to address the root causes of acne. These scams usually come in the form of a pill or some kind of "inner cleansing" regime. However, acne is a very complex condition, and can't be cured so easily.

Having suffered from acne for over twenty years, thoroughly researching the subject and looking for a cure, I have a pretty good idea of what the causes are. I can break them down to the following:

- **Genetics**
- **Personality**
- **Lifestyle**

There are also specific acne causes in adult women, which I will talk about later in this chapter.

Genetics

The main reason you get acne is genetics. My parents both suffered from some acne in the past, though never as severe as I had. However, genetically I do have a tendency towards acne.

There is scientific evidence that the chance of someone getting acne increases significantly if a parent or sibling had/has the condition. This would explain why, despite having the same lifestyle as your friends, they may have clear skin while yours is covered in lesions. They can eat and drink what they want, smear grease over their face and body, scratch and irritate their skin, go without sleep for 3 days, and still never get so much as a pimple.

Coming from the north of Scotland, I have a combination of Celtic and Nordic genes, so my skin is fair and sensitive. I take care not to stay in the sun for too long (not usually a problem in Scotland!) as my skin burns easily. My skin also suffers badly when I get an insect bite, triggering an inflammatory response, which results in a sore usually visible for weeks. Other triggers, such as stress, could theoretically cause inflammation that damages the walls of the skin's pores in people with sensitive skin, resulting in acne.

We are largely a product of our DNA, but the good news is that genes can, and do, express the information held in your DNA in different ways, so even if you have a tendency towards acne, it isn't inevitable and it CAN be controlled.

Skin Colour Considerations

The treatment for acne is the same for people of all colours. However, non-Caucasian people should take extra care when choosing an appropriate scar treatment, due to problems such as skin pigmentation. More information is available about scar treatments later in this guide.

All non-Caucasian peoples tend to suffer more from *hyperpigmentation* than white people. This is the appearance of dark marks on the skin after spots have healed. The marks may take many months to disappear. Topical (applied to the skin) retinoid drugs and hydroquinone (a skin lightening product) are common treatments for this problem, though the use of the latter is now banned or limited in many countries due to it being recognised as potentially cancer causing. What's more, many skin lightening products on the market can make acne worse. Use of a good UVA and UVB blocking sunscreen can help control hyperpigmentation in the first place.

Please note: do not use retinoids or hydroquinone if you are using benzoyl peroxide to treat acne.

White people tend to suffer from more cystic acne than people with darker skin. Also, acne is more apparent in lighter skin tones.

Asian people, especially East Asian women, often favour the use of skin lightening products containing ingredients such as hydroquinone. Some of these preparations can irritate the skin and cause acne. Asian people in general are more prone to *keloid* scarring than white people.

Keloids are red/purple coloured formations of scar tissue caused by excessive collagen production. Treatment options for keloids are outlined later in the guide.

Black people are less prone to deep cysts, but are prone to keloid scar formation. Black people should also take care choosing which hair products they use, as some products which black people commonly use contain ingredients that can block pores and cause acne.

Please note: the antibiotic Minocycline should not be taken by people of African descent as they are often hypersensitive to the drug.

References

delGiudice, P, & Yves, P. 2002. The widespread use of skin lightening creams in Senegal: a persistent public health problem in West Africa.*International Journal of Dermatology*. 41 (2), 69-72.

Goulden, V., McGeown, C.H. & Cunliffe, W.J. 1999. The familial risk of adult acne: a comparison between first-degree relatives of affected and unaffected individuals. *British Journal of Dermatology,* 141 (2), 297-300.

Halder, R.M.&Nootheti, P.K. 2003. Ethnic skin disorders overview.*Journal of the American Academy of Dermatology.*48 (Suppl 6), 143-8.

Poli, F. 2007. Acne on pigmented skin.*International Journal of Dermatology*. 46 (Suppl 1), 39-41.

Shah, S.K.& Alexis, A.F. 2010.Acne in skin of color: Practical approaches to treatment. *Journal of Dermatological Treatment*. 21(3), 206-211.

United States Food and Drug Administration. 2006. □Skin bleaching drug products for over-the-counter product use; proposed rule □(report). 1978N-0065. Available at: http://www.fda.gov/OHRMS/DOCKETS/98fr/78n-0065-npr0003.pdf (accessed 5th March 2017).

Personality

Acne is a very visible condition and the psychological effects can be devastating. It is commonly associated with the following psychological problems:

- ### *Low self-esteem*

Many acne sufferers lose confidence in themselves and find it hard even to make eye contact with people.

- ### *Social withdrawal*

Many of us hide away when we are having a particularly bad acne day. We cancel nights out, call in sick at work and skip school. Those of us who suffer from body acne also may avoid sports like swimming, where our skin is under the public's gaze. Relationship building can also be a problem, and we often become increasingly isolated.

• *Depression*

Those of us who have had acne for many months or years often develop a feeling of hopelessness related to the disease. We become more and more focussed on our skin and lose interest in hobbies and other activities. We often hate to look at ourselves in the mirror, and when we do, we see another spot erupting, which plunges us into deeper despair. Many develop sleep problems, feelings of apathy and worthlessness - all classic symptoms of depression.

• *Body Dysmorphic Disorder (BDD)*

This is a mental health problem where we become obsessed with our appearance. We may focus on an imagined defect or focus on a minor defect (such as a pimple) out of proportion to its severity. We constantly check our appearance in reflective surfaces such as shop windows or mobile phone screens. The sufferer often thinks they are ugly, even if they are actually not. The acne sufferer may not just think his skin is bad, but may also think he/she has other defects too, for example big ears. BDD can lead to social withdrawal, plastic surgery and even suicidal thoughts.

These are all commonly recognised psychological *effects* of acne, but our personality influences the severity and duration of the acne problem. Along with your DNA, your childhood experiences have largely determined the person you are today. Our mood changes, our habits change, and our behaviour changes depending on the social situation we are in, but our core personality remains pretty constant all our life. Psychologists classify the five core dimensions of personality as:

1. Openness

Characteristics of imagination and interest.

2. Conscientiousness

Attention to detail, thoughtfulness and organisation.

3. Neuroticism

Tendency towards anxiety and moodiness.

4. Extraversion

Degree of sociability, expressiveness.

5. Agreeableness

Qualities such as kindness and affection.

Research has shown that certain personality traits, particularly a high degree of neuroticism, can cause ailments such as asthma and stomach ulcers. It also suggests that people with anxious personalities double their chance of getting ill. This could logically include formation of acne.

In my experience, people with bad skin tend to display a lot of anxiety. Often they are sensitive types with a high sense of responsibility. Their feeling of self-worth is often low, making them susceptible to stress.

Of course, much of this could be a result of the acne itself - cause and effect are difficult to differentiate here - but our core personality probably does affect the condition of our skin. Our upbringing shapes our character; perhaps unhappy childhood experiences lead to a personality that causes the person to continue to suffer from acne long after others have freed themselves from the problem.

References

Friedman, H.S. & Booth-Kewley, S. 1987. The disease-prone personality: A meta-analytic view of the construct. *American Psychologist*, 42 (6), 539–555.

McCrae, R.R.& Costa, P.T. 1987. Validation of the five-factor model of personality across instruments and observers. *Journal of Personality and Social Psychology* 52 (1), 81–90.

Lifestyle

We can't change our DNA, and our personality is generally fixed from our early years, but, unless you are a monk or a soldier engaged in military combat, you do have control over the way you lead your life. In this section, I will discuss the role of the following in acne development:

- **Diet**
- **Stress**
- **Sexual Activity**
- **Sunlight**

- **Alcohol**
- **Exercise**
- **Clothing**

Diet

"You are what you eat".

Victor Lindlahr, American nutritionist, 1897-1969.

So the saying goes. The acne we get must be a result of the food we put in our mouths, right? Not according to every doctor and dermatologist I've ever seen. Time and time again I've been told acne is nothing to do with what you eat.

The reason is probably two studies published in the 1960's and 70's. These studies concluded that there was no link between chocolate consumption and acne. For some unknown reason, doctors took this as evidence for *all foods*, which is without doubt a very unscientific and unbelievable generalisation.

Since then, the medical community generally hasn't changed its tune. This is despite other research showing that there *is a link*, particularly with consumption of refined carbohydrates such as sugar and white flour. For example, one study showed that acne only emerged in a native Arctic community after they started to eat these refined foods. Unsurprisingly, they also started to develop higher rates of heart disease and diabetes.

I have spent over twenty years avoiding foods on my quest to be acne free, looking for that one ingredient that might just be the cause of my problem. In reality, the cause of acne is much more complex than that, but like many acne sufferers, I have always been convinced that there is a link between what I eat and the state of my skin.

I have previously eliminated: dairy products; eggs; wheat products; peanuts; corn; broccoli; cauliflower; barley; pineapples; oranges; kiwi fruit; spicy food; watermelon; cola drinks; kelp; and soy products. As you can probably imagine, this has caused me, and my family, all sorts of stress over the years. Constantly hearing people say "Oh, he doesn't eat that", having to scan ingredients labels, avoiding dinner invitations… the list goes on and on. However, most of it was unnecessary. Below is a list of foods that research and/or my personal experience has shown can cause/increase acne.

- **High Glycemic Load foods**

Glycemic Load (GL) (or Glycemic Index) represents the rate of carbohydrate absorption in the gut. This can also be considered the insulin raising potential of food, due to increased blood sugar levels.

The essential hormone insulin, which type 1 diabetes sufferers lack, has been linked to an increase in androgen production and an increase in skin cell turnover, both of which are factors in the formation of acne.

High GL foods cause a spike in blood sugar and insulin levels. These foods include pizza, sugary drinks, watermelon, white rice, over ripe bananas, sweets and bagels. Personally, eating too much of some of these foods, like white rice, doesn't seem to affect my skin at all. But whenever I eat too much sweet food, including fruit, I have some inflammation of existing acne, and more spots will usually appear a day or two later.

- **Kelp**

Kelp is a kind of seaweed which is rich in the trace element iodine. It is essential that we get enough iodine from our diet, but eating too many foods rich in the nutrient has been linked with - though not proven to cause - a type of acne called *acneiform,* which appears very quickly after ingestion of these foods.

My body does seem to have a negative reaction whenever I eat a lot of kelp. Acneiform produces pustules on parts of the body not usually affected, such as the belly and arms. However, it is very unlikely that iodine alone is the cause of your acne problem.

- **Spicy food**

Although there is no evidence linking these foods with increased acne, I usually get an outbreak on and around the nose if I eat a lot of spicy food such as chili peppers. This could be due to the sweat produced by the body's reaction to the chemical capsaicin, which is present in chilis. Sweat can irritate sensitive skin.

Many people are convinced that **food allergies** cause acne. Several years ago I sent a small sample of my blood to a famous lab for allergy analysis. They measured so called "IgG antibodies" in my blood, which are supposed to be the result of a reaction to certain foods, and indicative of food allergy. Two weeks later, I received my report, which stated that I had an allergy to dairy products, cola drinks and kiwi fruit.

So began ten years of avoiding these foods, with no improvement in my symptoms. In fact it probably did more harm than good, as I was always underweight during that period.

So do food allergies exist? Yes, but you will certainly know about it, as the symptoms will express themselves immediately, usually things like skin rash, wheezing, hives and, most seriously, anaphylactic shock. As for food allergies and acne, I couldn't find any scientific evidence supporting any link. Furthermore, I suffer from hay fever in the summer months, and I have never had a noticeable increase in acne at that time, despite the increase in antibodies.

There is much talk these days of food "intolerance", which is an interesting concept. This is a delayed reaction, up to several days after eating a suspected food. It may be possible that an increase in antibodies could cause an inflammation leading to acne several days later, but again, I couldn't find any hard scientific evidence for this. Conditions such as Irritable Bowel Syndrome (IBS) are affected by different foods, however, so if you feel uncomfortable after eating a certain food, then avoid it.

Overall, what you eat can have an effect on your skin, but many of the claims linking different foods with acne are just not true. Eating a healthy, balanced diet is the best advice. It may not cure your acne problem, but it will ensure you look the best you can every day. The last thing you want to do is to worry too much about what you put in your mouth. The stress and anxiety caused by this is likely to affect your skin more than the food itself. I will discuss the important role of stress in acne formation next.

References

Anderson, P. 1971. Foods as the cause of acne. *American Family Physician*, 3 (3), 102-3.

Fulton, J., Plewig, G.,&Kligman, A. 1969. Effect of chocolate on acne vulgaris.*The Journal of the American Medical Association*, 210 (11), 2071-2074.

Harrell, BL. & Rudolph, AH. 1976. Kelp diet: A cause of acneiform eruption. *Archives of Dermatology,* 112 (4), 560[letter].

Kristiansen, S., Endoh, A., Casson, P., Buster, J., & Hornsby, P. 1997. Induction of steroidogenic enzyme genes by insulin and IGF-I in cultured adult human adrenocortical cells. *Steroids*, 62 (2),258–65.

Powell, D., Suwanichkul, A., Cubbage, M., DePaolis, L., Snuggs, M. & Lee, P. 1991. Insulin inhibits transcription of the human gene for insulin-like growth factor-binding protein-1. *Journal of Biological Chemistry,*266 (28), 18868–18876.

Schaefer, O. 1971.When the Eskimo comes to town.*Nutrition Today*, 6 (6), 8-16.

Smith, R. & Mann, N. 2007. Acne in adolescence: A role for nutrition? *Nutrition and Dietetics,* 64, (Suppl 4), 147-149.

Stress

Other than genetics, stress is the main reason people get acne. By stress, I mean the feeling of being under excessive mental and/or emotional and/or physical pressure.

Common causes of stress are having a demanding job, relationship problems, and money problems. Other causes include excessive physical exercise, worrying about an upcoming event, and low self-esteem. Of course, acne itself can be a major cause of stress, so that many of us become trapped in a vicious cycle of stress, anxiety, and acne.

One man's stress, however, is another man's motivation. How we deal with pressures depends on the personality of the individual in question. Stress can be *chronic* (long term) or *acute* (short term), and result in both physical and emotional symptoms.

- **Acute stress**

This results in "fight or flight" responses such as increased heart rate and sweating. Acute stress can be beneficial, for example it can help give us focus before an important exam.

- **Chronic stress**

Chronic stress has no benefits, often leading to problems such as high blood pressure, sleep problems and depression.

Anxiety is a result of *stressors*. The stressor can be something like the appearance of a new spot overnight. We often worry about how our skin will appear in the morning when we look in the mirror. We may ask ourselves "Has that pizza I ate last night had any effect? How many new spots will there be?"

In the past, whenever I saw a new lesion had appeared, I could literally feel a wave of anxiety course through me. I started to understand that this feeling usually created even more acne, so I took steps not to study my skin too much. Whenever I obsess over my appearance, there is always an increase in acne a day or two later.

Acne also used to make me anxious and self-conscious in social situations. I always noticed an increase in skin oiliness at these times, and, again, acne a day or two later. These kind of feelings lead to problems of chronic anxiety and stress, which place a large burden on your physical and emotional state.

The scientific evidence linking stress with acne is strong. One study involving both male and female university students, showed a strong correlation between feelings of stress at exam times and severity of acne. Other research showed an increase in the number of acne lesions in interviewees following a particularly stressful interview situation.

Stress has also been correlated with slower healing of wounds in general. One study found that people who experienced high stress while caring for sick relatives showed slower wound healing than a control group.

So how does all this work? Why does stress lead to acne?

- Stress stimulates the body's adrenal glands into producing *androgens*, which can lead to extra sebum production.

- The hormone *cortisol*, again released by the adrenal glands, may also contribute to acne. Although cortisol is usually beneficial, for example in our "fight or flight" responses, chronically elevated levels of the hormone can be harmful. One effect of cortisol is to increase blood sugar levels, which can lead to increased acne. People with Cushing's disease, which causes sufferers to produce too much cortisol, often have - among many other symptoms - severe acne.

- Other studies link stress to *cell production* and *inflammation*. Research has shown that a molecule called *Substance P*, elicited by stress, can increase skin cell production and cause inflammation of the sebaceous glands, both of which are contributing factors in acne formation.

The processes and feedback mechanisms linking stress and personality with acne are complex, but there is no doubt that the severity of acne is closely related to the stress levels of the sufferer. Dealing with stress and anxiety are vital parts of acne management. I will explore techniques that will enable you to do this later in the guide.

References

Chiu, A., Chon, S.Y. &Kimbal, A.B. 2003. The Response of Skin Disease to Stress: Changes in the Severity of Acne Vulgaris as Affected by Examination Stress. *Archives of Dermatology,* 139 (7), 897-900

Kiecolt-Glaser, J.K., Marucha, P.T., Malarkey, W.B., Mercado, A.M. & Glaser, R. 1995. Slowing of wound healing by psychological stress. *Lancet,* 346 (8984), 1194- 1196.

Lee W.J., Jung, H.D.,Lee, H.J., Kim, B.S., Lee, S.J.& Kim do, W. 2008. Influence of substance-P on cultured sebocytes. *Archives of Dermatological Research,* 300 (6), 311-316.

Lorenz, T., Graham, D.T. & Wolf, S. 1953. The relation of life stress and emotions to human sebum secretion and to the mechanism of acne vulgaris. *Journal of Laboratory and Clinical Medicine,* 41 (1), 11-28.

Mayo Clinic. 2013. Chronic stress puts your health at risk. Available at: http://www.mayoclinic.com/health/stress/sr00001 (accessed 5th March 2017).

Morohashi, M. & Toyoda, M. 2001.Pathogenesis of Acne.*Medical Electron Microscopy*, 34 (1), 29-40.

Sexual Activity

The health benefits of safe, regular sex include lower blood pressure, lower stress levels, and a stronger immune system. However, don't overdo it! Sex more than two or three times a week has been linked to lower immunity.

Research suggests that sex and other forms of tender human contact can have a positive effect on your skin. Teenage boys often hear the old wives' tale that masturbation will give you spots. Is there any truth in this? Probably not. Actually, in one study on Chinese men, levels of testosterone peaked on the 7th day of sexual abstinence, and then declined. This shows a link between sexual activity and androgens. My conclusion from this is that abstaining from sexual activity could cause *more* acne, due to the increase in these hormones.

Simple hugging and kissing may also reduce acne symptoms. This could be due to the hormones *oxytocin* (the so called "love hormone") and *vasopressin*. One study found that arm blisters healed faster after tender human interaction, when levels of these hormones increased. It is believed that oxytocin and vasopressin can control the level of molecules called *cytokines* which cause inflammation.

References

Brody, S. 2006. Blood pressure reactivity to stress is better for people who recently had penile-vaginal intercourse than for people who had other or no sexual activity. *Biological Psychology*, 71 (2), 214-22.

Charnetski, CJ., Brennan, FX. 2004. Sexual frequency and salivary immunoglobulin A (IgA). *Psychology Report*, 94 (3, part 1), 839-44.

Gouin, JP., Carter, S., Pournajafi-Nazarloo, H., Glaser ,R., Malarkey, WB., Loving, TJ., Stowell, J. & Kiecolt-Glaser, JK. 2010. Marital Behavior, Oxytocin, Vasopressin, and Wound Healing. *Psychoneuroendocrinology*, 35 (7), 1082–1090.

Jiang, M., Xin, J., Zou, Q. &Shen J.W. 2003.A research on the relationship between ejaculation and serum testosterone level in men. *Journal of Zhejiang University. Science,* 4 (2), 236-240.

Sunlight

Sunlight is important for health, as it synthesises vitamin D in the skin. Of course, it can also lift our mood when we're feeling down.

Many people think that the sun can clear acne, but actually all it does is darken the skin so that it tones in with the colour of existing spots. Spending more than 20 minutes a day in the sun will damage your skin. In my experience, the typical result of sunburn is delayed acne a week or two later. The severity of the acne is usually worse than before the sun exposure, so my advice is to try and limit your daily time in the sun or use a good UVA and UVB blocking *non-comedogenic* (a product that doesn't block the skin's pores) sunscreen.

Reference

Gfesser, M., & Worret, Wl. 1996. Seasonal Variations in the Severity of Acne Vulgaris. *International Journal of Dermatology,* 35 (2), 116-7.

Alcohol

I first got acne around the time I started to go to pubs. For young British men like I was, going to a bar usually involves drinking a pint of lager as quickly as possible before moving on to the next place and repeating the process. Pub crawls can be great fun, and a good way to unwind, but we all know the negative effects drinking too much alcohol can have, from liver cirrhosis to high blood pressure and diabetes.

Although there is no scientific evidence linking alcohol consumption with acne, I am convinced that excessive drinking does make the problem worse. There are several reasons for this:

> 1.   Although most alcoholic drinks have a low *glycemic load*, some sweet beers, such as real ales, can increase insulin levels which may lead to acne.

> 2.   If you are drunk, you may be harsh on your skin when you wash, or even forget to wash completely, causing irritation.

> 3.   Your sleep will be disrupted if you drink alcohol, messing with hormone levels.

I haven't drunk alcohol for several years now, and although I suffered from acne for a couple of years after I stopped, I know I would find it very difficult to stay acne free if I went back to my old binge drinking ways. Having a social drink now and again is fine; just don't overdo it if you want acne free skin.

Exercise

Exercise is an integral part of a healthy lifestyle. Among other things, it can reduce stress levels, help you to lose weight and reduce your risk of getting seriously ill. However, too much is bad for your health, resulting in physical stress, and the problems that stress can cause. Athletes with intensive training regimes, for example, are prone to throat infections due to lowered immunity levels.

Personally, aerobic exercise such as running or cycling, has never increased my acne symptoms. However, whenever I have done weight training, my skin has suffered in the following days. This may be due to increased testosterone levels, which some scientific research (mainly on men) suggests may temporarily increase after exercising with weights.

Excessive sweating during exercise can cause skin irritation, so try to shower soon after your exercise regime if possible, then apply any skin product you may be using.

One final point: the benefits of exercise far outweigh the negatives. Like many other things regarding acne control, just don't overdo it!

References

Mackinnon, L.T. 1997. Immunity in athletes. *International Journal of Sports Medicine,*18 (Suppl. 1), 62–68.

Marin, D. P., Figueira, A. J. Jr., &Pinto, L. G. 2006. One session of resistance training may increase serum testosterone and triiodetironine in young men? *Medicine and Science in Sports and Exercise,* 38 (5) 285.

Schwab, R., Johnson, G. O., Housh, T. J., Kinder, J. E., & Weir, J. P. 1993. Acute effects of different intensities of weight lifting on serum testosterone. *Medicine and Science in Sports and Exercise* 25 (12) 1381-1385.

Clothing

Repeated pressure or friction on the skin such as from shirt collars, musical instruments or tight fitting shirts can cause a type of acne called *Acne Mechanica*. Symptoms are usually worse in hot weather. In my experience, continued irritation usually causes the spots to develop into cysts.

My worst affected areas were the back of the neck (due to shirt collars) and the shoulders (due to wearing a backpack). I used to often wear a backpack for long hours climbing mountains. The friction from the backpack combined with heat and sweat would really irritate my skin and cause back and shoulder acne.

If you can't eliminate the source of irritation, then wear a loose fitting cotton T-shirt next to the skin, try to shower as soon as you get home and follow the treatment advice later in the guide. This should help you manage to control the problem.

<u>*Acne in Adult Women*</u>

When adult women suffer from acne it is often a sign of changing hormone levels, particularly the hormones *progesterone* and *oestrogen*.

- Increased incidence of acne is often reported in the first three months of **pregnancy,** then again shortly after delivery of the baby. Usually the acne will disappear after a few months. The sufferer needs to take extra care treating acne during this time as acne treatments such as Accutane can harm unborn children.

- Some women also suffer from acne at **menopause**, decades after they stopped worrying about the issue. The problem should subside as hormone levels balance out, though again the treatment method later in the guide will help control any outbreaks you may have.

- 66% of women with acne reported a worsening of symptoms in the days leading up to **menstruation**. Traditional treatment options for this include low dose birth control pills, but the methods that I will outline later in the book will work well, and come without worrying side effects.

- Women with **Polycystic Ovary Syndrome** (PCOS) have high levels of androgens in their body, which often results in acne, as well as symptoms like increased body hair. Weight loss can reduce symptoms of PCOS somewhat, and oral contraceptives may also be prescribed.

Cosmetics

Acne caused by make-up is called **acne cosmetica.** Using the wrong cosmetics often traps women into a cycle of more make-up and more acne. If you must use make-up, use light, sheer, oil-free, non-comedogenic products and apply very lightly. Also, regularly wash brushes and so on. With the exception of eye make-up you should be able to remove make-up using water, a liquid cleanser and your bare hands. If not, the make-up is too heavy.

Please note: do not use wipes or napkins to remove cosmetics as this can irritate the skin.

References

Dunaif, A., Segal, K., Futterweit, W. & Dobrjansky, A. 1989. Profound peripheral insulin resistance independent of obesity in polycystic ovary syndrome. *Diabetes,* 38 (9) 1165–74.

Ebede, T.L., Arch, E.L. & Berson, D. 2009. Hormonal Treatment of Acne in Women. *The Journal of Clinical and Aesthetic Dermatology,* 2 (12) 16-22.

Honein, M.A., Paulozzi ,L.J. & Erickson J.D. 2001. Continued occurrence of Accutane-exposed pregnancies. *Teratology*. 64 (3) 142-147.

Lucky, A.W. 2004. Quantitative documentation of a premenstrual flare of facial acne in adult women. *Archives of Dermatology*, 140 (4) 423-424.

Singh,S., Mann, B.K., & Tiwary, N.K. 2013. Acne cosmetica revisited: a case-control study shows a dose-dependent inverse association between overall cosmetic use and post-adolescent acne. *Dermatology*, 226 (4).

2. Treatment Reviews

What follows is a guide to the treatments I tried in over twenty years of fighting acne. Some of them are commonly prescribed by physicians and dermatologists, others I bought over-the-counter or discovered online; on acne websites and in internet forums.

There are three main groups of treatments.

1. Prescribed Products

2. Over-The-Counter Products

3. Other Treatments

Disappointingly, and perhaps unsurprisingly, most so called acne "treatments" are totally ineffective. A whole industry has grown up around treating acne, with the sole aim of making profit at the expense of sufferers.

Many companies or websites use terms such as "holistic", "detox" or "miracle cure" when advertising their products or services. These terms should be viewed as red flags, warning you that the product or service is probably a total waste of your hard earned cash. "Detox" (or detoxification) for example is a word that is thrown about at will these days. The fact is that sweating or fasting won't expel any mysterious black evil substance from your body. Also, your liver and kidneys deal with toxic substances such as alcohol just fine. Although I wish there was, there is no "miracle" cure for acne, such as avoiding a certain food or popping a pill every morning. You will be free of acne, but only if you have some patience and are dedicated to the methods outlined later in this book.

Reference

Mayo Clinic. Do detox diets offer any health benefits? Available at: http://www.mayoclinic.com/health/detox-diets/AN01334 (Accessed 5th March 2017).

<u>Prescribed products</u>

• *Accutane (Isotretinoin)*

Accutane is probably the most well-known and controversial acne treatment available today. Since it entered the market in 1982, millions of severe acne sufferers have been prescribed the drug, usually after other treatments such as antibiotics have failed.

The Theory

Accutane works by reducing the amount of oil produced by the sebaceous glands, normalising the rate of skin cell production and reducing inflammation.

The drug takes time to work, with about 30% of patients reporting an *increase* in acne severity during the first month of treatment. However, after a few months, more than 90% of users have at least partial clearance of acne, most of them reporting no new acne lesions at all.

The majority of patients are permanently cured, with about a third reporting relapse, depending on the dose.

All this sounds wonderful, but the drug causes birth defects in pregnant women and has been linked to depression and suicide, though research regarding this has so far been inconclusive.

My Experience

I had my first course of Accutane when I was in my mid-twenties. In the UK, family doctors cannot prescribe the medicine, so I was referred to a dermatologist. The dose was 80 mg twice a day with food. This dose is regarded as high these days for someone whose body weight was only 70 kg. A typical dose now is 0.5-1.0 mg/kg body weight per day, up to 2 mg/kg for those with severe body acne. I was told to avoid prolonged exposure to sunlight, avoid Vitamin A supplements (Isotretinoin is a derivative of this vitamin), and to control alcohol consumption during my treatment period, which was 16 weeks.

During the first month my skin got much worse, with new spots appearing on my face, neck and chest. I also soon developed dry, chapped lips. Chapped lips are reported by most Accutane patients and the problem stayed with me throughout the treatment period, though the effect was lessened somewhat by regular application of lip balm.

Over the next few weeks my skin improved dramatically, with no new lesions coming through at all. Of course there was still scarring from old acne, which didn't seem to fade any faster while on the drug.

My skin continued to be acne free for the rest of the treatment, though strangely, I didn't particularly care. In fact while taking the drug, I was overcome by apathy, and had a constant heavy feeling in my head, like it was being gripped by a vice. I had thought I would be overjoyed when I finally managed to control my acne problem, but the reality was that I just felt tired and moody. Also, I developed pain in my lower back, and muscle pains, which got worse after exercise. These were symptoms that I would directly attribute to Accutane, as I hadn't experienced them before.

About six weeks after I stopped the drug, the first new acne lesion appeared, soon followed by many others, and my skin was just as bad as before. Four months later I started my second cycle of the drug. The pattern was repeated, with early worsening of acne followed by total clearance, and the same side effects, though the back pain was worse. When acne reappeared again a few weeks after I stopped treatment, I vowed never to take the drug again. The drug gave me so much hope, but failed me in the end.

Overall

All of the side effects I experienced are commonly reported by patients taking Accutane. Although most of the side effects disappeared soon after I stopped the treatment, to this day I still get some pain in my lower back.

This is my experience of using Accutane. Of course, there are many success stories, but I would strongly advise you to consider the side effects before embarking on a treatment programme.

References

Akman, A., Durusoy, C.,Senturk, M.,Kaya Koc, C., Soyturk, D &Alpsoy, E.2007. Treatment of acne vulgaris with intermittent and conventional isotretinoin: a randomized, controlled multicenter study. *Archives of Dermatological Research*, 299(10), 467-473.

Azoulay L.,Blais, L., Koren, G., LeLorier, J. &Bérard,A. 2008. Isotretinoin and the risk of depression in patients with acne vulgaris: a case-crossover study. *The Journal of Clinical Psychiatry*, 69(4), 526-532.

Demircay, Z., Kus, S. & Sur, H. 2008.Predictive factors for acne flare during isotretinoin treatment. *European Journal of Dermatology*, 18(4), 452-456.

Ellis, C.N. &Krach, K.J. 2001.Uses and complications of isotretinoin therapy.*Journal of American Academy of Dermatology*, 45(5), 150-157.

Ganceviciene, R.,&Zouboulis, C.C. 2009.Isotretinoin: state of the art treatment for acne vulgaris. *Journal of the German Society of Dermatology*, 8(Suppl 1), 47-59.

Mandekou-Lefaki, I.,Delli, F., Teknetzis, A., Euthimiadou, R. &Karakatsanis G.2003. Low-dose schema of isotretinoin in acne vulgaris. *International Journal of Clinical Pharmacological Research,*23(2-3), 41-46.

McLane, J. 2001. Analysis of common side effects of isotretinoin. *Journal of the American Academy of Dermatology,*45(5), 188-194.

Wysowski, D.K., Pitts, M. &Beitz, J. 2001.Depression and suicide in patients treated with isotretinoin (letter]. *The New England Journal of Medicine*, 344:460.

• *Adapalene*

The Theory

Adapalene is a retinoid (a chemical compound similar to Vitamin A) used as a topical gel or cream in acne treatment, in strengths of 0.1 and 0.3%. It is usually marketed under the brand name Differin®. Adapalene has a *comedolytic* effect on the skin (breaks down blackheads and opens up pores). It is also anti-inflammatory. Studies have shown that it reduces the number of lesions in acne sufferers.

My Experience

My doctor prescribed me 0.3% Differin® cream. I applied it to acne prone areas on the face, neck and upper body once a day, in the evening. As per the instructions, I was careful to limit my sun exposure while using the cream.

I had a small worsening of acne symptoms during the first two weeks on my face and neck, along with a little redness in the first week of application, but thereafter the cream worked quite well on these areas, reducing the number of pimples and cysts, but not clearing my skin. The treatment had no effect on the body acne.

I continued to use this product for about a year, with the same results. I had to pay many visits to the doctor during this time as the biggest tube is only 45 grams, which was only enough to last a couple of weeks, and few doctors in the UK will prescribe more than two or three tubes at a time.

Overall

Although, it didn't clear my skin, and had no effect on body acne, adapalene is one of the better treatments that I tried during my long battle with acne. However, there are better options.

References

Irby C., Yentzer, B. & Feldman, S. 2008. A review of adapalene in the treatment of acne vulgaris. *Journal of Adolescent Health,* 43(5), 421-424.

Tirado-Sánchez, A., Espíndola, Y.S., Ponce-Olivera, R.M. & Bonifaz, A. 2013. Efficacy and safety of adapalene gel 0.1% and 0.3% and tretinoin gel 0.05% for acne vulgaris: results of a single-center, randomized, double-blinded, placebo-controlled clinical trial on Mexican patients (skin type III-IV). *Journal of Cosmetic Dermatology*, 12(2), 103-107.

• *Antibiotics (Oral)*

This acne treatment has been around for decades, but oral antibiotics are still commonly prescribed by physicians for moderate acne cases.

The Theory

Excess sebum blocks skin follicles. P.acnes bacteria, loving the conditions inside the blocked follicle, multiply and cause inflammation. The result: spots. By killing the bacteria that cause the inflammation, antibiotics can clear the skin of spots.

My Experience

In the past, I have been prescribed **erythromycin**, and the tetracycline antibiotics **minocycline** and **doxycycline**.

The first oral antibiotic I tried was **erythromycin**, though these days it is only prescribed for topical application. My dose was 250mg twice a day. As with all antibiotics, I was told the drug would take time to work, even a few weeks. However, as the weeks passed, I could see no result, despite never missing a dose. My course of erythromycin ended after two months. I can't say I noticed any side effects, but my acne condition didn't improve at all, so for me the drug was a waste of time.

I had more success with **minocycline**. I was in my early thirties when I was prescribed the drug, as my acne problem had recently worsened again. The dose was 100mg once a day, before breakfast. As per the doctor's advice, I made sure I didn't take the medicine with milk or any calcium products. I had to have a blood test before taking the medicine, as the drug can interfere with liver function. I was also told it can cause discolouration of the teeth and skin. Needless to say, I started the treatment cycle with some apprehension.

By the third day, I noticed that I had no new spots. After two weeks, my skin was almost clear, with just some residual redness from old lesions. However, 6 weeks after starting on the drug, I woke one morning to find a cyst emerging on my neck. I felt totally deflated. Over the next two weeks, the acne came back with a vengeance and I was back where I had started two months before. Again, I didn't notice any side effects at the time.

I started **doxycycline** immediately after the minocycline course. The doctor prescribed me 100 mg twice a day for two months. Immediately the acne worsened and stayed bad throughout the treatment cycle. After that, I never took antibiotics for acne again.

Overall

So why did the antibiotics not help me? The answer is **antibiotic resistance**. Bacteria are constantly multiplying and creating new strains, with genetic mutations that make them resistant to certain antibiotics. This explains why minocycline was so successful for me at the beginning, then totally ineffective a few weeks later. This is a huge problem for effective antibiotic treatment of many diseases.

Though I had some short term success with minocycline, antibiotics did almost nothing for me. The usual story I hear from acne sufferers is that they work well for a short time, before the bacteria become resistant to the drug and the acne comes back again with a vengeance. Acne clearance commonly peaks around 6 weeks into an antibiotic treatment cycle, and then the drug becomes less effective, most patients returning to physicians with acne symptoms within 18 weeks of starting treatment.

Of the antibiotics commonly prescribed for acne, most research has shown minocycline to be the most effective, though it also has the most reported side effects. The most common side effects of antibiotics are diarrhoea, nausea and headaches. I didn't notice any of these while taking the drugs, but I have had some staining of the teeth in recent years, which lead me to have them professionally whitened - and I am not a smoker or a coffee drinker. I believe it is due to the minocycline.

Antibiotics are certainly not the cure for acne that many doctors would have you believe.

References

Leyden, J.J. & Del Rosso, J.Q. 2011. Oral antibiotic therapy for acne vulgaris: pharmacokinetic and pharmacodynamic perspectives. *Journal of Clinical and Aesthetic Dermatology,* 4(2), 40–47.

Ochsendorf, F. 2010. Minocycline in acne vulgaris: benefits and risks. *American Journal of Clinical Dermatology,* 11(5), 327-341.

Ozolins, M., Eady, E.A., Avery, A.J., Cunliffe, W.J., Po AL., O'Neill, C., Simpson, N.B., Walters, C.E., Carnegie, E., Lewis, J.B., Dada, J., Haynes, M., Williams, K. & Williams, H.C. 2004. Comparison of five antimicrobial regimens for treatment of mild to moderate inflammatory facial acne vulgaris in the community: randomised controlled trial. *Lancet,* 364(9452), 2188-95.

Ozolins, M., Eady, E.A., Avery, A., Cunliffe, W.J., O'Neill, C., Simpson, N.B. & Williams, H.C. 2005. Randomised controlled multiple treatment comparison to provide a cost-effectiveness rationale for the selection of antimicrobial therapy in acne. *Health Technology Assessment,* 9(1), iii-212.

Schafer, F., Fich, F., Lam, M., Gárate, C., Wozniak, A. & Garcia, P. 2013. Antimicrobial susceptibility and genetic characteristics of Propionibacterium acnes isolated from patients with acne. *International Journal Of Dermatology,* 52(4), 418-425.

Smith, K. & Leyden, J.J. 2005. Safety of doxycycline and minocycline: a systematic review. *Clinical Therapy,* 27(9) 1329-1342.

Over-the-counter (OTC) products

• ***Benzoyl Peroxide***

The Theory

Benzoyl Peroxide (BP) is a topical OTC or prescribed skin cream. The treatment has been around since the 1930s. Well known OTC products using BP include Neutrogena® On the Spot® and Clearasil® Daily Clear®. It is usually available in concentrations of 2.5% to 10%.

BP has, like adapalene, comedolytic properties but also has an antibacterial action. Unlike oral antibiotics, however, bacteria don't become resistant to BP, so it can be regarded as a long term acne treatment. Studies have shown BP to significantly reduce acne symptoms.

Common side effects experienced during treatment are skin peeling and reddening. BP can also bleach hair and clothes if care is not taken.

My Experience

I was first prescribed BP (brand name Brevoxyl®) by my doctor when I was a young university student. However, I didn't use the product correctly, and only applied it to existing lesions, thinking that the treatment would magically make them disappear overnight. Seeing no benefit in using the cream I gave up after a couple of weeks.

This is the common story I hear from acne sufferers regarding BP. Actually, a cure to my acne problem was right under my nose, so to speak. I just *didn't know how to use the product correctly*. What's more, most manufacturers don't tell you how!

After using a 2.5% concentration BP for a few weeks - more than twenty years after I first tried the treatment - *my skin was clear, and still is.* The key is:

1. To use lots of it.
2. To apply it twice a day to areas prone to acne.
3. To moisturise after application.
4. To be patient.

I will explain all this in more detail in the next chapter.

Overall

Used in the right way, BP is the most effective acne treatment we have today.

References

Harper, J. 2010. Benzoyl peroxide development, pharmacology, formulation and clinical uses in topical fixed combinations. *Journal of Drugs in Dermatology*, 8 (9), 482-487.

Mills, O.H., Kilgman, A.M., Pochi, P. & Comite, H. 1986. Comparing 2.5%, 5% and 10% benzoyl peroxide on inflammatory acne vulgaris. *International Journal of Dermatology*, 25 (10), 664–667.

Sagransky, M., Yentzer, B. & Feldman, S. 2009. Benzoyl peroxide: A review of its current use in the treatment of acne vulgaris. *Expert Opinion on Pharmacotherapy*, 10 (15), 2555-2562.

• *Maca Root (Lepidium meyenii)*

The Theory

Maca is a plant grown in the mountains of Peru. The root is used by native people as a vegetable and for its claims that it increases strength and virility, boosting sperm production. Some websites selling maca also claim that it can balance hormone levels and therefore alleviate acne. It is usually sold in powder form.

My Experience

I took 3 teaspoons of maca a day, mixed with water, for about three months. Although I quite enjoyed the taste, I noticed no other benefit, or any side effects, while taking the supplement.

Overall

Some clinical studies have credited maca - especially the black root variety - with increasing sperm production and semen volume. Levels of hormones, such as the androgens, didn't seem to be affected by taking the root. I could find no published research crediting maca root with lessening acne.

References

Gonzales, GF., Córdova, A., Vega, K., Chung, A., Villena, A. & Góñez, C. 2003. Effect of *Lepidiummeyenii* (Maca), a root with aphrodisiac and fertility-enhancing properties, on serum reproductive hormone levels in adult healthy men. *Journal of Endocrinoogyl*, 176 (1), 163–168.

Gonzales, G.F., Gonzales, C. & Gonzales-Castañeda, C. 2009. *Lepidiummeyenii* (Maca): a plant from the highlands of Peru--from tradition to science. *ForschKomplementmed*, 16(6), 373–80.

- ## *MSM (Methylsulfonylmethane)*

The Theory

This is another dietary supplement with big health benefit claims. The main one I saw on websites was that it relieves joint pain, but others include acne clearance and wrinkle reduction.

Websites selling the supplement state that our bodies are deficient in sulfur - which MSM is rich in - despite the fact that there is no Dietary Reference Intake (DRI) listed by the US National Academy of Sciences for this element.

My Experience

I took MSM in powder form, two teaspoons a day for six months. The result: no noticeable benefits or side effects.

Overall

The only benefit of taking MSM may be for reducing joint pain in people suffering osteoarthritis. Claims that MSM can clear acne are unsubstantiated.

References

Food and Nutrition Board, Institute of Medicine, National Academies. Dietary Reference Intakes (DRIs): Estimated Average Requirements. Available at: http://www.nationalacademies.org/hmd/Activities/Nutrition/SummaryDRIs/DRI-Tables.aspx (accessed 6th March 2017).

Kim, L.S., Axelrod, L.J., Howard, P., Buratovich, N. & Waters, R.F. 2006. Efficacy of methylsulfonylmethane (MSM) in osteoarthritis pain of the knee: A pilot clinical trial. *Osteoarthritis And Cartilage*, 14 (3), 286–294.

- ## *Probiotics and Prebiotics*

The Theory

Probiotics are live microbes -or more specifically, bacteria - which are purported to have many health benefits. The theory is that boosting the level of "friendly" bacteria in the gut improves microbial balance and therefore health. For this reason, many people also take them after a course of antibiotics.

Many strains of probiotics are available as tablets, capsules or powders, while some foods such as fermented yogurt, kimchi, and sauerkraut naturally contain them.

Prebiotics are claimed to be the food source of friendly bacteria, which can help them to flourish. Prebiotics come naturally in foods such as apples, or come in powder fibre form to be added to water.

The health claims of pre/probiotics warrant a book in themselves, so here I will just talk about the claims that pre/probiotics can help clear acne. Proponents of this theory often say that pre/probiotics do this by reducing the number of "toxins" in our bodies

My Experience

I took the probiotic *Lactobacilus Acidophilus* in capsule form twice a day. Each capsule was said to contain 5 billion "colony forming units", which I thought sounded impressive. I also took two tablespoons of prebiotic fibre in water twice a day before swallowing the capsules.

After six months, I could feel no effect from all this, except for the usual result of increased fibre intake: gas!

Overall

Some studies suggest a link between gut bacteria and acne, however, the US FDA hasn't approved any health claims up until now (6th March 2017). A joint UN and WHO report in 2001, supported claims that probiotics may have some benefits, particularly regarding gastrointestinal illness, but said that more research is needed. The same report also stated the importance of correct handling and storage of these live cultures, something to consider if buying them.

Summing up, probiotics may improve your health but won't cure your acne problem alone.

References

Al-Ghazzewi, F.H. & Tester, R.F. 2010. Effect of Konjac glucommanan hydrolysates and probiotics on the growth of the skin bacterium Propionibacterium acnes in vitro. *International Journal of Cosmetic Science*, 32 (2), 139-42.

Bowe, W. & Logan, A.C. 2011. Acne vulgaris, probiotics and the gut-brain-skin axis - back to the future? *Gut Pathogens*, 3(1).

Food And Agriculture Organization of The United Nations/World Health Organization. 2001. Health and nutritional properties of probiotics in food including powder milk with live lactic acid bacteria. *Report of a Joint FAO/WHO Expert Consultation on Evaluation of Health and Nutritional Properties of Probiotics in Food Including Powder Milk with Live Lactic Acid Bacteria, Cordoba, Argentina, 1-4 October 2001.*

Gibson, G.R. & Roberfroid, M.B. 1995. Dietary modulation of the human colonic microbiota: introducing the concept of prebiotics. *Journal of Nutrition,* 125(6), 1401–1412.

• *Salicylic Acid*

The Theory

This is a common ingredient of OTC acne products such as Oxy®, Proactiv® and Clearasil®, with strengths of between 0.5% and 2.0%.

Salicylic acid is a beta hydroxy acid, with *desmolytic* (exfoliates the skin, removing dead skin cells) and comedolytic effects. Studies have shown salicylic acid can be an effective treatment for mild to moderate acne, with minimal side effects at low concentrations such as those in acne products.

My Experience

Salicylic acid was the active ingredient in the first products I ever used; Clearasil® lotions, scrubs and cleansing pads. Lotions and pads I always used twice a day. None of these products helped me at all; actually the acne got worse. Scrubs cause irritation to acne prone skin, and in my opinion shouldn't be used.

Overall

Although it may be effective for mild acne cases, salicylic acid is not an effective treatment for people with moderate to severe acne.

References

Shalita, A.R. 1981. Treatment of mild and moderate acne vulgaris with salicylic acid in an alcohol-detergent vehicle, *Cutis*, 28(5), 556–561.

Shalita, A. 1989. Comparison of a salicylic acid cleanser and a benzoyl peroxide wash in treatment of acne vulgaris. *Clinical Therapeutics,* 11(2), 264-267.

- ## *Spirulina (Arthrospira platensis/Arthrospira maxima).*

The Theory

Spirulina is a type of cyanobacteria (blue green algae) often used to feed fish, and cultivated these days for use as a dietary supplement. Spirulina websites claim the supplement can boost the immune system, strengthen the nervous system and even treat liver disease. As for acne, spirulina is claimed to promote "skin metabolism" and consequently clear acne.

Usually it is sold in pill or powder form, but can also be bought for skin application as a cream. The claims seemed too good to ignore, so I gave the pills a try.

My Experience

I took three pills twice a day for six months. The effect was absolutely zero, except for a lightening of my wallet.

Overall

I could find no research crediting spirulina with acne reducing benefits, either topical spirulina or in pill/powder form. In fact, one study in the USA found that many marketed spirulina pills include contamination from a toxic blue green algae called *microcystin*, which has been linked with promoting tumours. Spirulina may do you more harm than good.

Reference

Gilroy, D., Kauffman, K., Hall, D., Huang, X., & Chu, F. 2000. Assessing potential health risks from microcystin toxins in blue-green algae dietary supplements. *Environmental Health Perspectives*, 108 (5) 435–439.

- ## *Vitamin B5 (Pantothenic Acid)*

The Theory

The Hong Kong doctor LH Leung published a paper in 1995 hypothesising that a lack of vitamin B5 in our bodies is the main cause of acne, and that super dosing with the vitamin will reduce sebum production and cure the problem. This is a common alternative choice for acne treatment these days and is big business online.

My Experience

I took 3 grams of Vitamin B5 daily in tablet form for three months. The DRI is only 5 *milli*grams per day, though research has shown that the vitamin isn't likely to be toxic in large doses such as I took. I saw absolutely no change in the condition of my skin during treatment with this supplement.

Overall

Dr Leung's hypothesis is merely that: a hypothesis. The study he conducted doesn't stand up to scrutiny; for example there was no control group used. There is no evidence that super dosing with Vitamin B5 can cure acne.

References

Leung, L.H. 1995. Pantothenic acid deficiency as the pathogenesis of acne vulgaris. *Medical Hypotheses*, 44(6), 490-2.

Trumbo, P. R. 2006. Pantothenic Acid. In Shils, M. E., Shike, M., Ross, A. C., Caballero, B. & Cousins, R. J. *Modern Nutrition in Health and Disease*. 10th ed. Philadelphia: Lippincott Williams & Wilkins. 462–467.

- ## *Vitamin C (Ascorbic Acid)*

The Theory

Vitamin C is essential for our bodies. It is an antioxidant and plays an important role in many bodily reactions, including collagen formation. As our bodies don't make the vitamin, we must source it from our diet. The DRI for adults is 60-75 mg/day, which we can get quite easily from a balanced diet, especially one that includes fruit and vegetables. A lack of vitamin C causes a disease called scurvy which can lead to death.

I came across reports on acne websites that high dosing with the vitamin may clear acne. The only published research on vitamin C and acne I could find dated from the 1950's, where the researcher found that dosing with 3 grams (3000 mg) of vitamin C a day lessened acne symptoms in most of the 53 sufferers. I decided to give it a try.

My Experience

I planned to take 1000mg of vitamin C three times a day, but on the first day, after taking the second pill, I felt very nauseous and had diarrhoea. I later found out that these are common symptoms of high dosing. I tried again the next day, but had the same problem, so lowered my dose to 3 * 500 mg pills a day, which I managed fine.

After six months, the acne symptoms hadn't changed, and I noticed no improvement in the rate of scar healing, so I stopped the treatment and just took vitamin C as part of a multivitamin pill, about 68mg/day. I can't say I noticed a difference in my skin condition or my overall health afterwards.

Overall

Adequate intake of vitamin C is essential for our health, but super dosing with the vitamin is problematic and doesn't seem to alleviate acne symptoms.

References

Morris, G. 1954. Use of vitamin C in acne vulgaris. *Archives of Dermatology and Syphilology,* 70 (3), 363-364.

Padayatty, S.J., Katz, A., Wang, Y., Eck, P., Kwon, O., Lee, J.H., Chen, S., Corpe, C., Dutta, A., Dutta, S.K. & Levine, M. 2003. Vitamin C as an antioxidant: evaluation of its role in disease prevention. *Journal of the American College of Nutrition,* 22 (1), 18–35.

World Health Organization. 1973. Toxicological evaluation of some food additives including anticaking agents, antimicrobials, antioxidants, emulsifiers and thickening agents. World Health Organization, 53(A), 1-520.

- *Zinc*

The Theory

Zinc is a trace element that is essential to our bodies. Among many bodily functions, it has roles in reproductive organ growth and gene expression. Zinc also plays a role in wound healing and has an anti-inflammatory effect on the body. Studies have shown that it can reduce acne severity.

My Experience

A study showed positive results on acne with a **zinc gluconate** supplement of 30mg per day, so that is what I chose. Zinc has several compounds, zinc oxide being the least absorbed of them, with studies tending to recommend zinc gluconate or glycinate for acne treatment. High doses of the element over 100 mg per day are toxic and can interfere with copper absorption and compromise immunity. Even 30 mg a day could reduce copper absorption, so I chose a supplement including this trace element.

I made the mistake of taking my first pill before breakfast and suffered nausea for about half an hour. Zinc tablets should never be taken on an empty stomach. I can't say I noticed any change in my acne symptoms in the years that I took this dose of zinc. These days I just take it as part of a mineral supplement, about 15.0 mg per day, and my skin is clear.

Overall

Zinc is an essential part of body and skin health so it is important that you get enough in your diet. I personally didn't benefit from a high dose, but it does seem to reduce acne symptoms in some people.

References

Allen, Lindsay H. 1998. Zinc and micronutrient supplements for children. *American Journal of Clinical Nutrition*, 68 (2 Suppl) , 495S-498S.

Berdanier, C. D., Dwyer, J.T. & Feldman, E.B. 2007. *Handbook of Nutrition and Food.* Boca Raton, Florida: CRC Press.

Decker, A & Graber, E.M. 2012. Over-the-counter acne treatments: a review. *Journal of Clinical and Aesthetic Dermatology*, 5 (5), 32–40.

DiSilvestro, R.A. & Swan, M. 2008. Comparison of Four Commercially Available Zinc Supplements for Performance in a Zinc Tolerance Test. *The FASEB Journal*, 22, (Suppl), 693.3.

Dreno, B., Moyse, D,, Alirezai, M., Amblard, P., Auffret, N., Beylot, C., Bodokh, I., Chivot, M., Daniel, F., Humbert, P., Meynadier, J. & Poli, F. 2001. Multicenter, randomized, comparative, double-blind controlled clinical trial of the safety and efficacy of zinc gluconate versus minocycline hydrochloride in the treatment of inflammatory acne vulgaris. *Dermatology*, 203 (2), 135–140.

Fosmire, G. J. 1990. Zinc toxicity. *American Journal of Clinical Nutrition*, 51 (2), 225–227.

Tan, H.H. 2004. Topical antibacterial treatments for acne vulgaris. *American Journal of Clinical Dermatology*, 5 (2), 79–84.

Other Treatments

- ## *Detoxification/Fasting*

The Theory

"Detoxification" (or "detox") is a widely used term these days, usually pertaining to some kind of elimination diet, fasting or "internal cleansing" regime, though sometimes to all of these at the same time. The "toxins" that advocates refer to are usually vaguely alluded to, but tend to include unspecified pesticides and air pollutants.

A whole host of books, internet guides and even TV shows have sprung up around the highly profitable subject of detoxification, often written or hosted by quack doctors with highly suspect medical qualifications, and sometimes endorsed by celebrities. Benefits of detox claimed on various websites and guides include stress reduction, weight loss, improved energy levels and even protection against cancer. A common claim is that detoxing can cure acne. Most advocates of detox, but not all, do advise consulting with your doctor before embarking on any detoxification programme.

My Experience

I stumbled across a popular online website and was impressed by its guarantee that I would have clear skin in

30-60 days. I paid about $30 US, and downloaded a guide as well as a host of free bonus attachments promoting the benefits of "healing water" and so on.

Following the programme wasn't simple, however. It includes "parasite cleanses" "liver flushes", and extensive supplementation. All this means a lot of time and monetary investment. Products required include wormwood (for the parasite cleanses), and olive leaf extract (as a supplement), but there are many, many more. The fasts were particularly difficult, just eating apples and cucumbers for three days, in preparation for "liver flushes" where I had to drink olive oil mixed with lemon juice (vomit inducing).

During the first two weeks, my skin improved, appearing less oily, with less acne than before. After six weeks, my skin was still somewhat better than before I started the regime, but my weight had dropped by 14 pounds, and I had very little energy. I had already been thin at the start of the programme, now I looked skeletal. In fact, it took me several years to put the weight back on again. My skin was better, but, with the weight loss, *I looked worse.* I had to stop this regime before it had serious consequences for my health.

Overall

I could find no scientific research explaining why my skin showed some improvement during the regime. It is probably because of low blood sugar and insulin levels due to fasting. Despite this, we *need adequate food to survive.* We cannot fast forever. In fact, other than eventual death by starvation, this kind of detox regime could be harmful to our bodies. Coffee enemas, for example, have been associated with cases of colitis and septicaemia.

As for "detoxification" in general, the only medically recognised definition of the word is for the treatment of people withdrawing from substance abuse, which is unrelated to the kind of detoxification spouted by quacks and alternative medicine practitioners. I could find no peer reviewed scientific evidence supporting any of the claims made about detox diets and so on. The reduction in acne symptoms that I had was down to starvation, not "detox". As one leading Australian doctor concluded in an article about the subject, "presently, detox is more of a sales pitch than a science".

References

Berg, J.M., Tymoczko, J.L & Stryer, L. 2002. *Biochemistry (5th edition)*. New York: W H Freeman. Section 30.3.

Cohen, M. 2007. 'Detox': science or sales pitch? *Australian Family Physician*, 36 (12), 1009-1010.

Mishori, R., Otubu, A. & Jones, A.A. 2011. The dangers of colon cleansing. *Journal of Family Practice*, 60 (8), 454-6.

Tan, M.P. & Cheong, D.M. 1999. Life-threatening perineal gangrene from rectal perforation following colonic hydrotherapy: a case report. *Annals of the Academy of Medicine, Singapore*, 28 (4), 583-585.

3. How To Be Acne Free

I recommend you read both The Product Free Method™ and The Product Method™ to find out which one is most suitable for you. The Product Free Method™ requires commitment and some degree of mental discipline. I advise you to try this method for a few weeks to see how it goes. However, don't expect immediate effects: raising your self-esteem for example can take time.

If you lack the willpower to stick with the plan, or find it too restrictive, then The Product Method**™** may be better suited to your needs. Please be aware that the advice given in The Product Free Method™ is useful for both.

RealAcneResults™ Method 1:

The Product Free Method™

Please note: a concise guide to this method is available in the appendices.

In summary: building self-esteem, reducing stress, and changing your lifestyle.

Please note: keep using the The Product Free Method™ even if your skin becomes totally clear. This is very important, as the acne will probably come back in a few days if you stop. With the exception of teenagers who may grow out of acne, both methods outlined in this guide are long term commitments for most people.

Building Self-Esteem

Low self-esteem is a common result of acne, but can also be a cause. It is a feeling of low self-worth, where we become blinded to any positive qualities we may have or any positive contributions we can make.

Many acne sufferers already had low self-esteem as children. When acne comes along it just makes the problem worse. Of course, many acne sufferers were perfectly happy and confident before they started to get acne, but they often become more withdrawn and start to obsess over the spots on their face and body, to the point of despair. These self-destructive thoughts cause stress and anxiety that can lead to more outbreaks. It is time to break the link between low self-esteem and acne.

Talking about feelings of low self-esteem with a registered psychotherapist is highly recommended if you suffer from this problem. I also recommend reading the book "Overcoming Low Self Esteem" by Dr Melanie Fennell of Oxford University, which uses Cognitive Behavioural Therapy techniques.

However, there are several things you can do to get a more positive and realistic view of yourself again without professional help. These techniques can also help with stress reduction.

- **Identify your *bottom line* and create a new one**

This is the heart of feelings of low self-esteem. Bottom lines are usually developed in childhood, but for many acne sufferers the bottom line is "I am ugly".

Bottom lines are often outdated opinions of yourself, or just plain wrong. People tend to develop biased thinking to maintain their bottom line. For example a man or woman rejects us so we presume it is because they think we are ugly. Actually it could be because they are married, or something else unrelated to our appearance.

Create a new bottom line, for example "I am an attractive person with lots to contribute to the world".

- **Challenge *rules for living***

Situations such as talking to an attractive woman or man may activate our bottom line and create anxious predictions e.g. that she/he will reject us.

This anxiety creates physical symptoms such as sweating. To deal with this, we develop rules for living. These keep us from activating our bottom line.

For example a man might avoid talking to an attractive woman, or practice what he is going to say again and again before approaching her. Rules for living actually make our feelings of low self-esteem worse. Identify and challenge them.

- **Make a list of everything you are good at, or were good at when you were younger**

Examples could include cooking, speaking a foreign language, playing computer games, helping people with personal problems, blowing bubbles with bubble-gum, or keeping a tidy desk at work. Make a point of reading the list every day.

- **Make a list of things you need to do every day**

Accomplishing goals, however small they may seem, is a great way to raise your self-esteem.

Every evening, write down a couple of things you want to accomplish the next day. This can be simple things such as writing an email to a friend you haven't contacted for a long time, or bigger tasks such as studying Chinese for two hours.

The feeling of completing your goals day after day should make you feel much better about yourself. If you don't accomplish them, don't be hard on yourself, but strive to do better next time.

- **Ask close friends what is attractive about you**

They may say something like your eyes, your sense of humour, or the way your nose creases when you laugh.

We often forget our positive attributes when we suffer from acne, but actually these can be far more noticeable to others than the acne itself. Having acne doesn't mean you are ugly! Write positive comments down and, again, read them every day.

- **Learn to identify negative thoughts, and stop them in their tracks**

For example, "what I say in this meeting is of no importance". Tell yourself it *is* important. Don't focus on negative things, such as the state of your skin. If your skin is in a bad state, obsessing over it in the mirror can lead to *cognitive distortions* where we think our appearance is worse than it really is. This will lower your self-esteem even more and create more anxiety, leading to more spots.

- ## Learn to say no to people

Those with low self-esteem are often scared of saying no in case they hurt others feelings or are rejected by them. The fact is that people don't respect "yes men", and anyway, the most important person is *you.*

- ## Reward yourself

Make sure you do something you enjoy every day, even it's just watching an episode of your favourite sitcom or having a glass of wine on a Saturday night. If you have had a particularly fulfilling day, or it's your birthday, buy yourself a gift as a way of congratulating yourself.

All this can take time, but stick with it and it will eventually pay dividends for your skin and for your life in general.

Reference

Fennell, M. 2009. *Overcoming Low Self-esteem: A Self-help Guide Using Cognitive Behavioral Techniques.* London: Constable & Robinson Ltd.

Reducing Stress and Anxiety

We know that stress can cause acne. The best way to deal with the problem of stress is to remove the reason you have the stress in the first place. For example getting out of an abusive relationship, quitting a high pressure job, or hiring a nanny to look after your screaming kids. However, this may be easier said than done, and is sometimes unrealistic.

Here I will present some advice to control stress levels so that your life can continue in a healthier and more attractive way.

- **Don't multitask**

Doing too many things at the same time not only raises stress levels but also reduces productivity. If you're writing a document, don't text and send email at the same time. Focus on the task at hand.

- **Nurture your relationships**

If you are in a romantic relationship, take time to appreciate your partner each day. Simple holding and kissing will reduce stress and increase levels of the inflammation reducing hormones oxytocin and vasopressin. A healthy sex life will also benefit you.

Compliment your friends and tell them how much you appreciate them. They may even return kind words to you, all of which fosters positive feelings and less stress.

Make sure you keep in touch with your friends. Having an active social life gives you a more realistic view of yourself, away from the self-criticism that can foster if we spend too much time alone. It also gives you a more relaxed all round attitude.

- **Exercise**

Studies have shown people who exercise regularly are less likely to suffer from depression than non-exercisers and are also more resilient to stress.

The biggest problem many people have is getting started. If this is a problem for you, try to approach exercise as a fun activity not something that you *must* do. Engaging in competitive sports such as tennis or football will increase your enjoyment as well as your social interaction, all while raising your heart rate.

Try to do moderate (such as mountain hiking or flat road cycling) to vigorous (e.g. aerobics, singles tennis, football) aerobic exercise three times a week for at least thirty minutes. But remember not to overdo it: exercising vigorously every day for example could cause you more harm than good.

Shower and put on clean clothes as soon as you can after exercise.

- **Meditate daily**

Meditation is no longer just the preserve of tree huggers, Buddhist monks and sixties rock stars. It is now a well-respected technique with benefits including stress and anxiety reduction and pain alleviation. Medical authorities such as Britain's National Health Service now employ it as a treatment option for these and other problems.

Well conducted scientific studies have contributed to this acceptance of a previously "alternative" treatment. For example, one Chinese study on 80 university students found that twenty minutes of daily Integrated Body Mind Training (IBMT) for only five days resulted in a drop in cortisol concentrations, along with a corresponding reduction in stress and anxiety levels compared to a control group.

IBMT is very similar to the technique I use called the **body scan**, focussing on breathing and awareness of the body. A transcript of this is outlined in Appendix 3 of this book.

- **Coping with anxiety**

You can use the breathing technique used in the body scan any time you feel anxious or stressed. For example, if you have an argument and feel angry, find a quiet place and focus on your breathing for a minute or two, filling your lungs with the relaxing colour and breathing out the negative colour you associate with.

This also helps if you feel you are having a bad skin day. Just imagine the breathing and the colour calming the acne and taking it away.

If you are sceptical about this at all, consider for a moment that research on "biofeedback" methods - which use instruments to measure bodily functions such as heart rate, skin temperature and muscle tension - has shown that we have the ability to control these normally involuntary bodily functions through sheer will, some of which can have a positive effect on the skin. The influence your mind can have on your skin should not be underestimated.

- **Get enough sleep**

We all know how touchy we feel if we don't get a good night's sleep. Even two hours less sleep per night reduces our resilience to stressful situations, increases blood cortisol levels and also our level of inflammatory molecules called cytokines.

I usually suffered a worsening of acne if I had even one night of deprived sleep. Not everyone needs eight hours sleep per night - personally I need between six and seven - but if you feel tired in the afternoon, then you are not getting enough at night. Just don't sleep all day!

References

Leproult, R., Copinschi, G., Buxton, O. & Van Cauter, E. 1997. Sleep loss results in an elevation of cortisol levels the next evening. *Sleep*, 20 (10), 865-870.

Rubinstein, J.S., Meyer, D.E & and Evans, J.E. 2001. Executive Control of Cognitive Processes in Task Switching. *Journal of Experimental Psychology - Human Perception and Performance*, 27 (4), 763-797.

Salmon, P. 2001. Effects of physical exercise on anxiety, depression, and sensitivity to stress: a unifying theory. *Clinical Psychology Review*, 21 (1), 33-61.

Shenefelt, P.D. 2003. Biofeedback, cognitive-behavioral methods, and hypnosis in dermatology: is it all in your mind? *Dermatologic Therapy,* 16 (2), 114-122.

Tang, Y.Y., Ma, Y., Wang, J., Fan, Y., Feng, S., Lu, Q., Yu, Q., Sui, D., Rothbart, M.K., Fan, M. & Posner, M.I. 2007. Short-term meditation training improves attention and self-regulation. *Proceedings of the National Academy of Sciences of the USA*, 104 (43), 17152-17156.

Vgontzas AN, Zoumakis E, Bixler EO, et al. Adverse effects of modest sleep restriction on sleepiness, performance, and inflammatory cytokines. *Journal of Clinical Endocrinology and Metabolism*. 2004;89:2119–2126.

Changing Your Lifestyle

The habits you have can have a big effect on your skin. Watching what you eat and drink, being careful how much sun exposure you get, reducing how often you touch your skin, cleansing properly, wearing the right clothes, and supplementing, all play a part in acne reduction.

- **Eat the right foods**

The best advice here is balance. Eating too much of any one food is not beneficial to your general health or the state of your skin. Try to eat a healthy diet rich in vegetables and whole-grains, with room for some meat, dairy or other protein source such as tofu or beans.

I tend to use sunflower oils or olive oil over animal fats or other oils. Personally, I try to eat whole wheat pasta and bread but can't stand brown rice: white rice doesn't cause me any problems.

For snacks, nuts and fruit are good options, but not too many of either. The occasional burger, chocolate bar or piece of cake is okay. Eliminating too much just causes stress. Also, don't keep eating until your stomach is full. This just leads to blood sugar spikes. Leave a little room at the end of your meal.

Limit consumption of sweet foods

It's okay to eat a little candy or birthday cake, but don't eat the whole chocolate bar. Just have a couple of pieces. Also don't eat too much fruit at one sitting. Pineapple, for example, has a very high sugar content.

Don't eat kelp

Kelp contains a lot of iodine which may lead to acne.

Limit consumption of spicy foods

Don't over-do it on the fiery burritos, Sichuan Hotpot or Chicken Madras. Try to stick to less spicy options when you're eating out.

- **Watch what you drink**

Drink a lot of water

Bottled or filtered water is generally recommended, though many places, for example my hometown in Scotland, have good quality water straight from the tap. Peppermint tea is great, especially in the evening.

Limit consumption of sweet drinks

This applies to fruit juice as well as soda. Go for the diet option if you have to.

Limit consumption of alcohol

A glass of wine is okay now and again.

Limit coffee and tea consumption

Caffeine is known to raise cortisol levels in the body, especially during times of stress, so don't pour yourself a double espresso when you're working to deadline on an important project. If drinking coffee, have decaf. Peppermint and fruit teas are great choices and are caffeine free.

- **Take care in the sun**

A little sun exposure every day is important, but in summer you need to take extra care not to get sunburn. If staying indoors isn't practical, then use a good SPF 30 or higher non-comedogenic UVA and UVB blocking sunscreen, and wear a hat. In tropical countries, you should take precautions all year round.

Also bear in mind that if you participate in winter activities such as skiing, UV rays can reflect from the snow surface causing your skin to burn. Wear a good sunscreen!

- **Limit touching your skin**

Touching your skin and picking at spots causes irritation leading to inflammation, more acne and scars. If you have this habit, *get out of it*. Wash your hands well before applying any skin creams, make-up or sunscreen, and *apply the product gently*.

- **Supplement**

Take 30mg a day of zinc gluconate or glyconate, with added copper. Split the dose into two pills, one after breakfast and one after dinner.

Take 25µg of Vitamin D_3 a day, as limiting your sun exposure and wearing sunscreen reduces your body's synthesis of this essential vitamin.

- **Cleanse**

You should try to shower after you get up and before you go to bed. This is particularly important for those with body acne. If this isn't possible, then at least try to shower in the evening.

If you build up a sweat during the day, for example during vigorous exercise, then it is advised to shower as soon as practical afterwards. Exercising before my morning shower works best for me.

When showering, use a gentle, non-comedogenic, cleanser on your skin and only wash the acne prone areas with your hands for a few seconds. *Do not rub or use a cloth.* You should then dry yourself gently with a towel, using dabbing motions, again taking care not to rub.

- **Be careful about clothing**

Wearing clothes that are too tight can aggravate your skin and cause acne mechanica. This is particularly the case for body and neck acne. If wearing a collared shirt, try to undo the top button and choose a soft cotton fabric.

Also, be careful about the laundry detergent you use. I find fabric softeners and strong detergents irritate my skin.

If you have body acne, then consider buying a bag you can carry rather than wearing a backpack. If you can't avoid this, then use The Product Method™, detailed in the next section of the guide, on your back and shoulders.

References

al'Absi, M. & Lovallo, W.R. 2004. Caffeine effects on the human stress axis. In: Nehlig, A. *Coffee, tea, chocolate and the brain*. Boca Raton, Florida: CRC Press. 113–31.

RealAcneResults™ Method 2:

The Product Method™

In summary: very effective results with less impact on your lifestyle.

If you follow the instructions as set out below, I am confident that the Product Method™ will give you acne free skin. After more than twenty years spent looking for a permanent solution to beating acne, experimenting with different products and regimes, I eventually found a solution in The Product Method™.

The method requires **patience**, **dedication** and the use of **several products**, but the payback is huge: acne free skin and a better life.   I recommend you follow the advice laid out in The Product Free Method™ too, as this will be beneficial to your general health and will reduce skin oiliness, but it is not essential.

The products you are required to use are widely available from drug-stores. However, they are slightly different depending on whether you suffer from just facial acne or have acne on your body and/or the back of your neck too. If you have body acne, you will need to use a lot of product. The good news is, there are manufacturers out there who can provide the products you need in big bottles.

Facial Acne Products:

Non-comedogenic liquid cleanser

Non-comedogenic moisturiser

2.5% Benzoyl Peroxide

Optional: jojoba oil

Body/Neck Acne Products:

Non-comedogenic liquid cleanser

Non-comedogenic moisturiser

2.5% Benzoyl Peroxide

10% Non-comedogenic Alpha Hydroxy Acid (Glycolic Acid)

Optional: jojoba oil

Before beginning the programme, you must read the following:

- ### Be patient

It may take a few weeks to see a major improvement in your skin. The acne on my face and neck began to clear up after two weeks, and was pretty much gone after six weeks. However, it took three months before my back and shoulders were clear. Please be patient as *the end result is worth it.*

- ### Expect some redness and peeling

During the first two to three weeks of treatment you will experience some facial redness and mild peeling as your skin adjusts to the products.

Personally, I got on with my life as normal, as the redness just resembled mild sunburn. Jojoba oil is great for applying on areas where the skin is peeling, and it is also non-comedogenic so won't cause new spots to form. Don't give up the treatment, however much you want to! The redness and peeling will subside. You will see results soon.

Please note: if you experience swelling, severe skin reddening or severe peeling, stop using the product and talk to your doctor. A small number of people are over-sensitive to BP.

- **You *must* moisturise**

It may go against your instinct, but moisturising is *essential* for the method to work. For some reason, most over-the-counter benzoyl peroxide product manufacturers do not tell you to moisturise. This is a huge oversight and results in overly irritated skin that causes many people to give up the treatment.

- **Existing scars will take time to fade**

Unfortunately, the method outlined here won't make existing marks and scars disappear any quicker, but it will prevent new acne lesions from forming in the first place.

- **Benzoyl Peroxide can bleach your clothes and hair**

I get around this by being very careful when applying the BP. This is especially true around the hairline. I also allow the products to dry first before putting on my clothes.

This works fine three seasons per year, but the heat of summer can make you sweat and cause bleaching. I tend to wear white clothes on my upper body in summer if I think sweating is going to be a problem that day, though grey also seems to be okay. Wearing a thin, cotton T-shirt next to your skin is also a good idea if you have a tendency to sweat a lot, as this will protect the outer layers.

Also be aware that BP can bleach towels and bed sheets, so choose colours wisely.

- **Keep using the Product Method™ even when your skin is clear.**

This is *very important*, as the acne will probably come back in a few days if you stop applying the products. With the exception of teenagers who may grow out of acne, both methods outlined in this guide are long term commitments for most people.

- **Discipline**

Don't miss an application. Even missing one morning or evening treatment can result in spots during the next few days. This is another reason why I recommend cutting down on alcohol, as applying the products is often the last thing you want to do when you are drunk.

- **You may need a third application.**

If you exercise and sweat profusely during the day, you should shower afterwards and apply the product again. To avoid having to do this, try to schedule exercise in the morning or in the evening an hour or two at most before you shower.

Facial Acne Method Steps.

Please note: a concise guide to this method is available in the appendices.

How often?

For the first week, once a day, in the morning. This allows your skin to get used to the BP. After that, twice a day, once in the morning and once in the evening, ideally around twelve hours between applications.

Please note: for men, do all this after you shave. Do not apply product to thickly bearded areas.

1. Cleanse

This can be done either in the shower, or at the sink. Firstly wet your face, then, using your hands, wash your face gently with the non-comedogenic cleanser for about ten seconds. Rinse with water until there is no cleanser left on your face. Dry gently with a soft towel, patting the towel on your face, *not* rubbing. **Do not use a cloth at any stage of the process**.

Wait about ten minutes for your skin to dry completely. This can be speeded up by a couple of minutes if you turn on a warm or cold (in summer) air fan a few feet away. Ten minutes may seem a long time, but I use this time to brush and floss my teeth and do other grooming.   The Product Method can improve other aspects of your appearance too!

2. Apply the 2.5% BP treatment

Firstly, wash and dry your hands well. For the first week only use a little BP, about ⅛ teaspoon/bean sized amount (0.5 ml, pictured below), a little more if you have acne on the front of the neck.

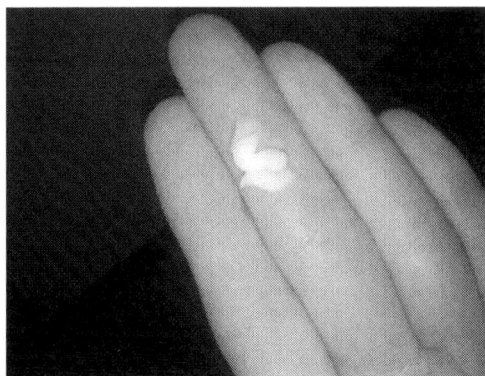

Up the amount at the end of the first week gradually to about a teaspoon/grape sized amount (4 ml, pictured below) by the end of week 3. This may seem a lot, but is **essential** to the effectiveness of the method.   A little more BP is okay. Don't use less.

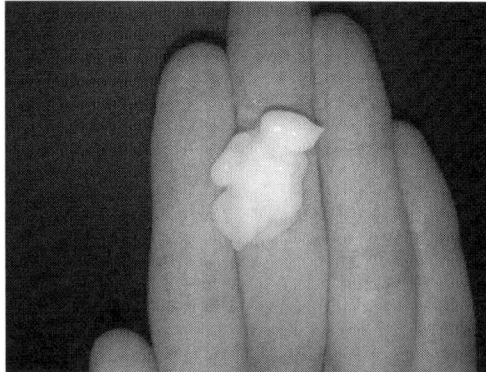

Gently spread the BP around your face, avoiding the sensitive area around the eyes. **Do not rub the BP in.** This should take no more than a minute or so. Wash and dry your hands.

Wait about ten minutes for the treatment to fully absorb into your skin. I use this time to meditate for a few minutes. Again, using a fan should speed up the process by a minute or two.

3. Moisturise

From the beginning of the treatment, use about a teaspoon/grape sized amount (4ml, see BP picture above) of non-comedogenic moisturiser, a little more if you also have acne on the front of your neck.

Gently spread the moisturiser gently around your face and neck. **Do not rub the moisturiser in**. Again this should take no more than a minute, and will take about ten minutes to fully absorb. Wash and dry your hands.

Body/Neck Acne Method Steps

The skin on the body and neck is generally thicker than on the face, and with larger pores. Acne on the back/side of the neck, and on the chest, shoulders and back is often nodulocystic in nature, taking longer to treat than facial acne.

The main difference in the treatment here is the use of **Glycolic Acid** in place of the general moisturiser on the body and back/sides of the neck. Glycolic Acid is an Alpha Hydroxy Acid (AHA). AHA has exfoliating properties and promotes collagen production, so is often used in "chemical peels" at 30% to 70% concentrations, and as an anti-ageing product in the beauty industry.

I suggest you use a concentration of no more than 10%. At this strength, the AHA will lightly exfoliate your skin, leaving it smoother, help the BP fight the acne, and also have a moisturising effect. I find it gives excellent results on the thicker skin on the back/side of the neck, chest, and the upper and lower back.

*Please note: it is vital that you **limit your sun exposure** and/or use a good quality UVA and UVB blocking sunscreen on any exposed skin that is being treated with AHA. You can mix a penny sized amount of sunscreen into the AHA before applying. If you stop using AHA, continue taking precautions for a week after discontinuation. AHA makes your skin very sensitive to the sun.*

After a few months of treatment, you can try a non-comedogenic moisturiser in place of the AHA, using the same quantity. This is a cheaper and more convenient option, which is effective for me. AHA, however, is a good ally at the beginning of the programme.

How often?

For the first week, once a day, in the morning. This allows your skin to get used to the BP and AHA. After that, twice a day, once in the morning and once in the evening, ideally around twelve hours between applications.

Please note: for men, even if you have substantial body hair, you should still apply product on these areas if they are prone to acne. Just take more care to apply product carefully.

1. Cleanse

This should be done in the shower. Firstly wet your face and body, then, using your hands, wash all acne prone areas gently with the non-comedogenic cleanser for no more than a total of one minute.

Rinse well until there is no cleanser left on your face or body. Dry gently with a soft towel, softly patting the towel on your face and body's acne prone areas, *not* rubbing. **Do not use a washcloth at any stage of the process**.

Wait about ten minutes for your skin to dry completely. This can be speeded up by a couple of minutes if you turn on a warm or cold (in summer) air fan a few feet away. Ten minutes may seem like a long time, but I use this time to brush and floss my teeth and do other personal grooming. The Product Method can improve other aspects of your appearance too!

2. Apply the 2.5% BP treatment

Remember, for the first week, only apply in the morning. Thereafter, apply twice daily.

Firstly wash and dry your hands well. If you get acne on the back and sides of the neck, use about a ½ teaspoon sized amount (2 ml, pictured below) of BP on these areas:

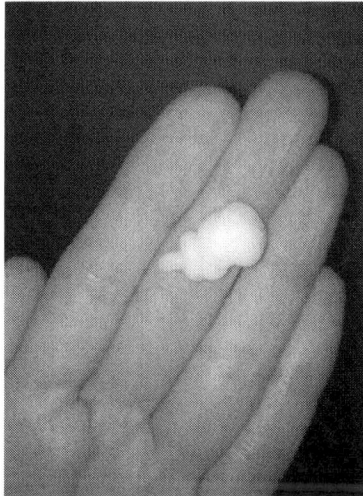

For the chest and upper back/shoulders, use about a teaspoon/grape sized amount (4 ml, pictured below) for each side:

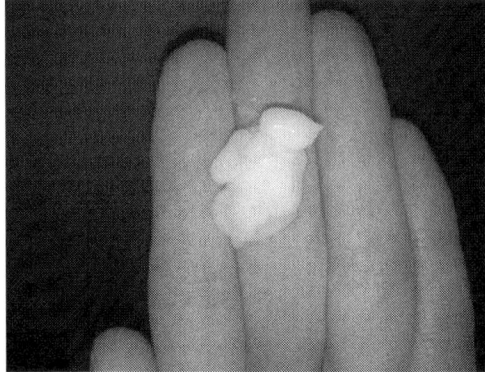

You may need a total of 4 teaspoons: one teaspoon for the left chest area, one teaspoon for the right chest, one teaspoon for the left back/shoulders and one teaspoon for the right back/shoulders. Use more if you get acne all the way down your back.

Gently spread the BP around the acne prone areas. **Do not rub the BP in**. This should take no more than two minutes to do. Wash and dry your hands.

Wait about ten minutes for the treatment to fully absorb into your skin. I use this time to meditate for a few minutes. Again, using a fan should speed up the process by a minute or two.

3. Apply the AHA

Remember, for the first week, only apply in the morning. Thereafter, apply twice daily. If you get acne on the back and sides of the neck, use

about a ½ teaspoon sized amount (2 ml - see BP picture above) of non-comedogenic AHA on these areas. For the chest and upper back/shoulders, use about a teaspoon sized amount (4 ml - see BP picture above) for each side.

You may need a total of 4 teaspoons: 1 teaspoon for the left chest area, 1 teaspoon for the right chest, 1 teaspoon for the left back/shoulders and 1 teaspoon for the right back/shoulders. Use more if you get acne all the way down your back.

Add a penny sized amount of sunscreen to the AHA for any areas that may be exposed to the sun.

Gently spread the AHA around the acne prone areas. **Do not rub the AHA in**. This should take no more than two minutes to do. Wash and dry your hands.

Wait a few minutes before putting on your shirt, in order to let the AHA fully absorb into your skin.

Remember, after a few months of using the AHA, you may want to change to a non-comedogenic moisturiser.

References

Decker, A & Graber, E.M. 2012. Over-the-counter acne treatments: a review. *Journal of Clinical and Aesthetic Dermatology*, 5(5), 32–40.

4. Staying Acne Free

Sometimes I feel lucky to have suffered from acne for so long. Most acne sufferers live a very healthy lifestyle, eating the right foods, drinking less alcohol and so on. However, we often lose focus on other aspects of our appearance such as our hair and our teeth. Now that your skin is looking good, you may also want to consider getting a new hairstyle, visiting the dentist or improving your daily grooming regime. All this can do wonders for your self-esteem. You may even be lucky enough for your friends to remark on how great you look!

But don't rest easy. Staying clear of acne is a long term commitment for most people. If you give up applying the methods as laid out in this guide, it is highly likely that the acne will return. Whichever of the two methods you use, **it *must* become part of your daily habits**, just like brushing your teeth twice a day is to everyone. Whether you are on holiday, on a business trip or a bachelor party weekend with your buddies, make sure you incorporate the treatment method into your schedule.

The payback is priceless. People have said to me that The Product Method™ is costly and time consuming. Maybe, but the benefits far outweigh these costs. For many people who suffered from acne, a whole new life opens up once they are clear. This is likely to benefit your personal relationships, your studies, your career... in fact almost every aspect of your life. A simple thing I now appreciate is having a massage every month. I would never have considered getting a massage when my acne symptoms were at their worst, but now I wonder how I managed without it.

So, stick with the method no matter how good your skin looks. **Don't become complacent**. Also, if you get the odd pimple, don't despair: I do too. This is normal: I hardly know anyone who doesn't get the odd spot or two now and again. The key point now is that *it's no big deal.* Having one or two spots is nothing compared to what you had before. You now have control over your appearance and won't hear whispered comments any more about your skin. Acne is no longer "*my* acne".

As time goes on, you will start to disassociate yourself from acne, and may start to at last do things you always wanted to do, but felt that acne stopped you from doing. That's fantastic, but **don't be complacent**. Your acne treatment should by then be a habit. You also may want to help others who suffer from this terrible condition. Be an agent for change in their lives.

One problem does remain, however, after the spots have gone: scarring. Time is a great healer, and my scars have gradually faded, but you may want to speed up the process. Next, I will go through the options available.

5. Acne Scars

There are two groups of acne scars: **depressed** and **elevated**.

Depressed (atrophic) scars

These are sometimes called "craters" and appear below the level of the rest of the skin. They are the most common type of acne scars and usually appear on the face, giving it a "pockmarked" appearance.

- **Ice-pick**

These are a series of small holes in the skin, hence the name "ice-pick".

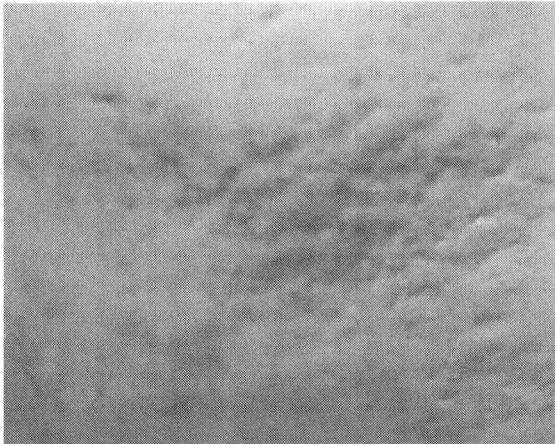

- **Boxcar**

These appear as larger holes than ice-pick scars, and have the appearance of small depressed squares.

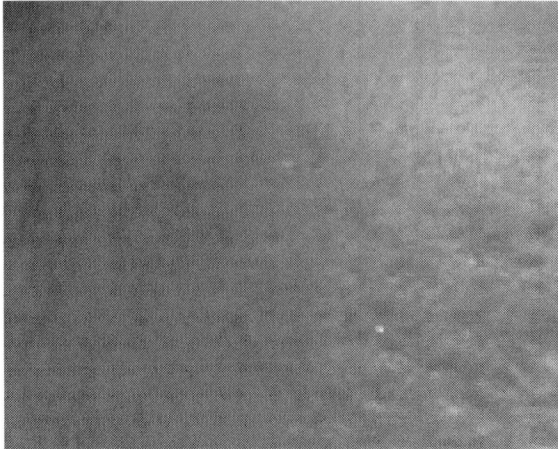

- **Rolling**

They have a wave like appearance, wide and shallow, giving the appearance of aged skin.

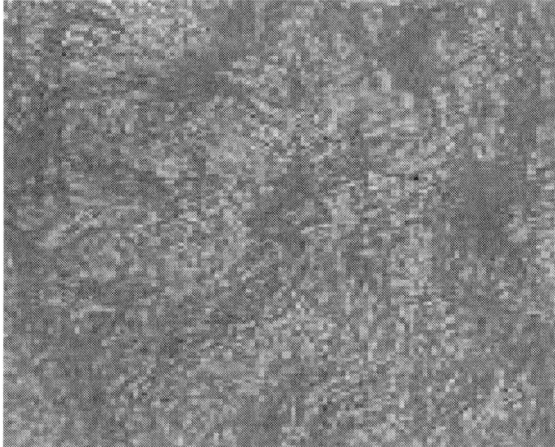

Elevated scars

These are a result of excessive deposit of collagen during the scar healing process. They are more common in people with dark skin and usually appear on the chest, back and shoulders, but occasionally on the face and neck. They are more difficult to treat than depressed scars.

- **Hypertrophic**

These are pink in colour and firm to the touch. They don't grow beyond the site of the original spot.

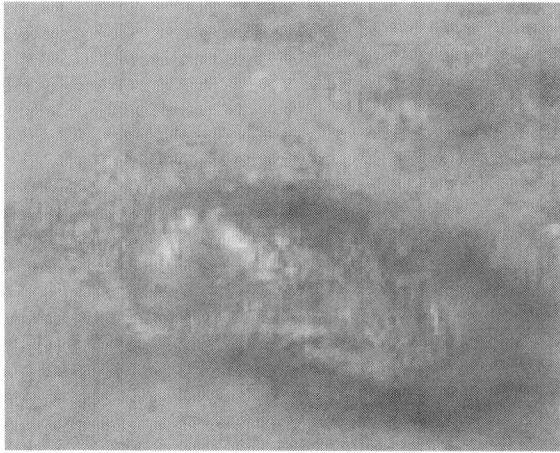

- **Keloid**

These scars are darker in colour than hypertrophic scars and form layers of collagen extending beyond the site of the original spot. They can grow to several centimetres in length.

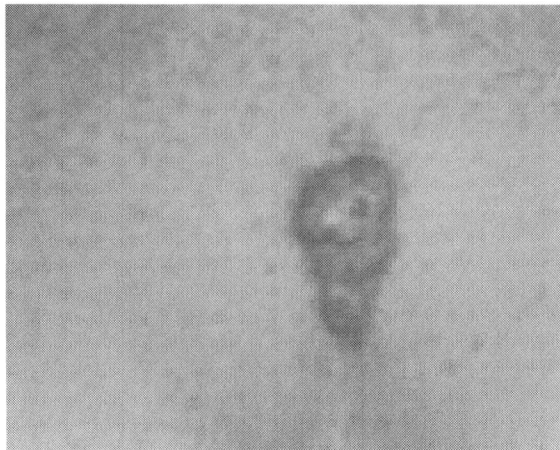

Reference

Fabbrocini, G., Annunziata, M.C., D'Arco, V., De Vita, V., Lodi, G., Mauriello, M.C., Pastore, F. & Monfrecola, G. 2010. Acne scars: Pathogenesis, classification and treatment. *Dermatology Research and Practice*, Volume 2010.

Scar Treatment Options

It goes without saying, that the best option is **prevention of acne**. The methods previously outlined in this guide should enable you to achieve this.

Please read the following advice before embarking on a course of treatment.

- Make sure you are well clear of new acne before treating any scars.

- Consult your doctor before embarking on any scar reduction programme (the exceptions are treatment using topical gels or silicone gels/sheets.)

- Take extra care if you are pregnant as some scar treatments can be dangerous for you and your unborn baby.

- Make sure that the surgeon who will perform any procedure is *certified,* and ask to see other patients' before/after photographs and testimonials. A reputable and competent surgeon should be able to advise you about all the methods below, and find the most suitable one/combination for your scarring situation.

- If you are using The Product Method™, then you must take extra care when considering which scar treatment method to opt for, as you may not be able to apply the products for a while after some scar procedures.

The only scar treatments I have personally tried are silicone sheeting, silicone gel and Contractubex® gel.

Depressed Scar Treatments

- **Chemical peels**

This treatment uses agents such as AHA at varying concentrations to reduce the appearance of acne scars, blotches and wrinkles. Peels are most effective at removing blotches. Repeat treatment sessions will be needed to improve the appearance of depressed scars.

Particularly for those with dark skin, extra care should be taken, as *hyper*pigmentation (darkening of skin) or - less commonly - *hypo*pigmentation (lightening of the skin) may take place. Other side effects may include skin flakiness and burning as well as increased sun sensitivity for people of all skin colours.

- **Dermabrasion/Microdermabrasion**

These techniques are generally used on the face for depressed scars. Dermabrasion is done under anaesthetic and removes the outer layer of skin (the epidermis), while microdermabrasion is more superficial. Dermabrasion is the more effective of the two, but neither method produces perfect results, and they can be expensive.

Side effects of these treatments can include hyperpigmentation and hypopigmentation (again especially in darker skinned individuals) and infection. **If you have taken Accutane within the previous 6 months, do not use these methods.**

- **Punch techniques**

These involve surgically removing or loosening the depressed scar and either suturing the wound or replacing it with skin from another part of the body. These techniques work well in combination with laser resurfacing, particularly on ice pick and small boxcar scars. However, reported side effects of punch techniques include keloid formation.

- **Laser treatments**

These techniques are generally *ablative* or *non-ablative*. I will also talk about *fractional* laser treatments.

Ablative laser techniques.

These work by melting, vaporising or evaporating the scar tissue, usually with CO_2 or Erbium YAG lasers. Up to 80% improvement in scar appearance has been reported using CO_2 lasers. Candidates for laser treatment should have been acne free and not used Accutane for at least one year. They should also have no history of keloid scars. Ablative treatments have many possible side effects, and are very expensive, especially if follow up treatment is required.

Recovery time can take several weeks, particularly for CO_2 ablation, with dressings having to be worn for a few days after treatment. Fungal infections, hyperpigmentation, hypopigmentation and hypertrophic scarring have been reported, the risk of scarring increasing after over-aggressive treatment.

Non-ablative techniques

These have less side effects, but also less impressive results on acne scars. They stimulate collagen production and skin tightening through the use of infra-red lasers.

Fractional Photothermolysis (FP)

This is a recent technique that only focusses on small fractions of the skin, creating microscopic thermal wounds.

Ablative Fractional Resurfacing

This combines FP with ablative CO_2 laser treatment, resulting in fewer side effects than the latter method alone, but higher effectiveness than just FP. Several treatments are usually required, with eventual costs running into the thousands of US dollars. Like all laser techniques, it can take months to see the full benefit of the treatment.

- **Needling**

A sterile needling tool is run across acne scarred areas, in order to stimulate collagen production. Repeat treatments are needed - usually about three - and full effects will take about a year to become apparent. The treatment is quite effective on depressed scars and has less risk of skin pigmentation than techniques such as dermabrasion.

- **Augmentation**

With this technique, filler material is injected into the depressed scar. Fat is often used as it has less side effects than injecting materials such as silicone, which can cause skin ulceration and bumpiness among other things. Fat is generally transplanted from the thigh or buttocks area to the scar, though about 50% will be reabsorbed into the body after a year. The cost is cheaper than laser surgery, but positive results are inconsistent, with the best results being on rolling scars.

- **Subcision**

The scar is cut away allowing blood clots underneath to form new tissue, levelling the skin surface. This may take several treatment sessions, though costs are lower than methods such as laser treatment. There is usually bruising for two weeks after treatment, and side effects can include reappearance of the scar, and hypertrophic scarring. Subcision works well in combination with other therapies, a combination of peeling, subcision and fractional laser methods being quite effective, with 55% improvement of the scars on average after one year.

Which Treatment Option Should I Choose For Depressed Scars?

If you have the money to pay for it, and can stand the recovery time, then I would suggest a combination of FP and ablative CO_2 laser treatment (Ablative Fractional Resurfacing). This is a good option for people of all skin colours, as the risk of pigmentation is lower than ablative treatment alone.

In my opinion, none of the cheaper options are particularly effective.

Please note: if you are using The Product Method™, then you shouldn't apply any product on scar treatment areas until the skin has totally healed from the procedure(s).

References

Chandrashekar, B. & Nandini, A. 2010. Acne scar subcision. *Journal of Cutaneous and Aesthetic Surgery*. 3(2), 125-126.

Ellenbogen, R. 1990. Invited comment on autologous fat injection. *Annals of Plastic Surgery*, 24, 297.

Fabbrocini, G., Annunziata, M.C., D'Arco, V., De Vita, V., Lodi, G., Mauriello, M.C., Pastore, F. & Monfrecola, G. 2010. Acne scars: Pathogenesis, classification and treatment. *Dermatology Research and Practice*, Volume 2010.

Grevelink, J.M. & White, V.R. 1998. Concurrent use of laser skin resurfacing and punch excision in the treatment of facial acne scarring. *Dermatologic Surgery*, 24(5), 527–530.

Hantash, B.M., Bedi, V.P., Kapadia, B., Rahman, Z., Jiang, K, Tanner, H., Chan, K.F. & Zachary, C.B. 2007. In vivo histological evaluation of a novel ablative fractional resurfacing device. *Lasers in Surgery and Medicine*, 39(2), 96–107.

Kang, W.H, Kim, Y.J., Pyo, W.S., Park, S.J. & Kim, J.H. 2009. Atrophic acne scar treatment using triple combination therapy: dot peeling, subcision and fractional laser. *Journal of Cosmetic and Laser Therapy*, 11(4), 212–215.

Elevated Scar Treatments

The general rule is that the older the scar is, the more difficult it will be to control and reduce in size.

- **Steroid therapy**

Injection of steroids is a common way to treat keloid and hypertrophic scars. The steroids stop collagen production and act as an anti-inflammatory agent, reducing the size of the scars and the discomfort felt. The treatment is affordable and there is no recovery time, though several treatments may be necessary before significant improvement is seen, and there is a chance of the scar coming back. Reported side effects include skin pigmentation and infection, and the injections are said to be quite painful. Greater success may be seen when combined with the cryotherapy method, which also reduces the pain of the steroid injections.

- **Cryotherapy**

Liquid nitrogen is applied to the scar, freezing it and causing the scar tissue to die off. Repeat treatments are usually needed. The technique is generally used on body scars due to the risk of facial disfigurement, as side effects include blistering and skin pigmentation. The treatment is usually quite effective, typically reducing the height of keloids by over 50% after two treatment sessions, and it also works well in combination with steroid injections.

- **Silicone treatments**

These are available in tubes of **gel** for direct topical application on elevated scars, or in the form of silicone **gel sheets** to apply as a dressing on top of the scars. Silicone works by promoting hydration into the scar and also by adding increased pressure onto the scar. It is important to note that it could take months to notice any difference in the appearance of old elevated scars using gel or sheeting.

Silicone gel sheeting

This has been used as a scar treatment since the early 1980's and studies have shown it has some effectiveness on keloids and hypertrophic scars.

I used Cica-Care® silicone gel sheeting for about six months. The sheet has to be cut into pieces that stick onto the scar. The silicone pieces can be reused but must be cleaned twice daily before they are re-applied. I noticed a little improvement in the hypertrophic scars during the treatment, but nothing like what I expected. The improvement was about 20% at most. I gave up using this method due to the inconvenience of application. If you have only one or two scars to treat, then it is worth trying silicone sheeting, but other methods are probably more effective.

Silicone gel

One study of this showed a 50% reduction in hypertrophic scar thickness after eight weeks of twice daily application.

I used Dermatix® silicone gel for about a year, applying it twice a day on the hypertrophic scars. Although it was much more convenient to use than the sheeting, I didn't notice any improvement in the scars. Also, the gel can be quite expensive, though I got it on prescription from the British NHS, which reduced the cost somewhat.

- **Other Topical Gels**

The pharmaceutical company Merz, market two products Mederma® and Contractubex® that they claim can improve the appearance of elevated scars.

Mederma® gel contains the active ingredient *allium cepa,* which is extracted from onions.

Contractubex® gel includes the active ingredients *heparin* and *allantoin,* as well as onion extract. Studies on Contractubex® show improvement in hypertrophic scars after a few months of use, but mainly in lightening the colour of the scar, not in reducing the overall size. *It should be pointed out that the studies were not based on scars resulting from acne.*

I used Contractubex® gel twice a day on hypertrophic scars for about two years. There was some improvement in the appearance of the scars, though this also occurred on ones that I did not apply the gel to. In my opinion, time is a greater healer than the gel itself.

- **Pulsed Dye Laser**

This recent laser treatment has been shown in studies to significantly reduce the size of elevated scars. It works by contracting blood vessels and loosening the collagen fibres in the scar tissue. Two or three treatments may be required. Scars tend not to grow back, though reported side effects include skin pigmentation, so the treatment is best recommended for people with light skin. The treatment is expensive if you have many scars to treat, but it is definitely an option worth considering.

Please note: other types of laser surgery are not recommended as treatments for elevated scars, as scar recurrence is common.

- **Cytotoxic Injections**

Fluorouracil and Bleomycin are drugs which are usually used in chemotherapy for cancer patients, but which are increasingly being used as a treatment for elevated scars. Studies have shown good results in flattening keloids and hypertrophic scars after repeat treatment sessions with either of these drugs, sometimes completely flattening the scar, even scars over 18 months old. One study showed that a combination treatment of fluorouracil with steroid injections and pulsed dye laser gave even better results. As with other injections used in scar treatment, skin pigmentation can be a side effect.

Please note: *women should not use this treatment if they are pregnant.*

Which Treatment Option Should I Choose for Elevated Scars?

Although none of the methods are perfect, there are some good choices these days for keloid and hypertrophic scar treatment.

For people with lighter skin, I would suggest pulsed dye laser as the best treatment option, possibly in combination with cytotoxic and steroid injections if you don't mind the discomfort, though all this could be expensive if you have many scars to treat. It is also a consideration for people with ethnic skin if your scars are confined to the body, as any pigmentation that may occur will be less conspicuous. Otherwise, you could consider using silicone gel sheeting, especially if your scars are not too old or numerous.

Please note: if you are using The Product Method™, take care not to apply product on treated areas during any scar treatment recovery period. If you use the silicone sheeting or silicone gel scar treatment, you can keep applying the BP and moisturiser/AHA around these areas as normal.

References

Alster, T.S. 1997. Laser treatment of hypertrophic scars, keloids, and striae. *Dermatologic Clinics,* 15(3), 419-429.

Bodokh, I. & Brun, P. 1996. Traitement des chéloïdes par infiltrations de Bléomycine. *Annales de Dermatologie et de Vénéréologie,*123(12),791-794.

Fabbrocini, G., Annunziata, M.C., D'Arco, V., De Vita, V., Lodi, G., Mauriello, M.C., Pastore, F. & Monfrecola, G. 2010. Acne scars: Pathogenesis, classification and treatment. *Dermatology Research and Practice*, Volume 2010.

Fitzpatrick, R. E. 1999. Treatment of inflamed hypertrophic scars using intralesional 5-FU. *Dermatololgic Surgery*, 25(3), 224-232.

Hosnuter, M., Payasli, C., Isikdemir, A. & Tekerekoglu, B. 2007. The effects of onion extract on hypertrophic and keloid scars. *The Journal of Wound Care*, 16(6), 251-254.

Mustoe, T.A., Cooter, R.D., Gold, M.H., Hobbs, F.D., Ramelet, A.A., Shakespeare, P.G., Stella, M., Téot, L., Wood, F.M. & Ziegler, U.E. International Advisory Panel on Scar Management. 2002. International clinical recommendations on scar management. *Plastic and Reconstructive Surgery*, 110(2), 560–571.

Nemeth, A.J. 1993. Keloids and hypertrophic scars. *Journal of Dermatologic Surgery and Oncology*, 19(8), 738–746.

6. Products You Can Use

Below is a list of products that you can use with confidence in acne treatment and prevention. I have used all of these products at one time or another with positive results.

Please note: I have no affiliation with any companies or individuals who manufacture, sell or distribute these products.

Benzoyl Peroxide

- **Neutrogena® On The Spot® Acne Treatment**

This is an effective 2.5% BP cream. However, it only comes in 21 ml (0.75 fl oz.) tubes, which isn't convenient for people with a large area of skin to treat.

- **Acne.org® Benzoyl Peroxide Treatment**

The main advantage of this BP gel is that it comes in 59 ml (2 fl oz.) 236 ml (8 fl oz.) and super large 472ml (16 fl oz.) bottles. It is also very cost effective compared to other BP products on the market, and applies very nicely indeed. However, Acne.org® products are only available online, so you must pay a delivery charge outside the U.S.

Moisturisers

- **Cetaphil® Moisturizing Lotion**

This non-comedogenic moisturiser is quite light and easy to apply. It comes in 59 ml (2 fl oz) 118 ml (4 fl oz) 236 ml (8 fl oz) and 532 ml (16 fl oz.) bottles. Widely available.

- **CeraVe® Moisturising Lotion**

This is a non-comedogenic lotion available in 236 ml (8 fl oz.) 354 ml (12 fl oz.) and super large 531 ml (18 fl oz.) bottles. It feels less greasy than some other moisturisers, however contains parabens.

Alpha Hydroxy Acid

- **Acne.org® AHA⁺**

Once again, Acne.org® comes up trumps with this easy to apply product. Like most of their other products in comes in 59 ml (2 fl oz.) 236 ml (8 fl oz.) and super large 472ml (16 fl oz.) containers. It is also quite cost effective. It is a yellow colour, which might not appeal to everyone.

- **Alpha Hydrox® AHA Soufflé**

This 10% AHA moisturises well, but only comes in a 50 ml tub (1.7 fl oz.).

Liquid Cleansers

- **Cetaphil® Gentle Skin Cleanser Wash**

This non-comedogenic cleanser is widely available and comes in convenient 59 ml (2 fl oz.), 236 ml (8 fl oz.), 472 ml (16 fl oz.) and 590 ml (20 fl oz.) containers. It doesn't lather, so isn't a suitable choice for a shaving foam.

- **Acne.org® Cleanser**

Available in 59 ml (2 fl oz.) 236 ml (8 fl oz.) and 472ml (16 oz.) bottles, this non-comedogenic cleanser foams well, which makes it a good option for use as a shaving foam.

Jojoba Oil

This oil comes from the seed of the jojoba tree, which grows in the desert of Mexico and the south-western United States. It is a wonderful ally for people who are prone to acne, as it is non-comedogenic and moisturising. As well as applying it to my skin, I also use it to moisturise my lips. I find a little dab of this oil also calms down pimples on the odd occasion when I get one.

- **Acne.org® Jojoba Oil**

This comes in a 236 ml (8 fl oz.) bottle. The 100% jojoba oil is organic and certified.

- **Desert Essence® 100% Pure Jojoba Oil**

Desert Essence® produces 60 ml (2 fl oz.) and 118 ml (4 fl oz.) sized bottles of jojoba oil. An organic option is available.

Sunscreen

For your face, you should apply about a ¼ teaspoon of sunscreen to get enough protection. You can also mix it with your moisturiser before applying.

- **Neutrogena® Ultra Sheer® Dry Touch Sunscreen**

This sunblock is light, easy to apply, and is non-comedogenic. It blocks both UVA and UVB rays and is available in a range of SPFs, from SPF 30 to SPF 100+ in an 88 ml (3 fl oz.) bottle. Widely available.

Concealers

- **Almay® Clear Complexion™ Concealer Corrector**

This little gem of a 5.3 ml (0.18 fl oz.) tube goes a long way. Apply a tiny drop to your finger, and smooth out before applying lightly to any red areas. It won't block your pores, and comes in different shades. It is available in selected retailers and also online.

- **Neutrogena® Skin Clearing® Blemish Concealer**

A good back up if you can't find the Almay® concealer, this cover stick is oil free, non-comedogenic, and widely available. The size is 1.4 g (0.05 fl oz.) and it comes in a range of shades.

Shaving Products

I use Taylor of Old Bond Street® Shaving Cream, which is luxurious and just fantastic. It can be ordered online. Gillette® Series® shaving foam for sensitive skin is widely available and does just fine. Also, a silvertip badger shaving brush is indispensable for me pre-shave. For a blade, I use a Gillette® Mach 3®.

Don't douse your face and neck with cologne after shaving. One of the moisturisers used in The Product Method™ will do the trick for soothing your skin.

Appendix 1.The Product Free Method™-Concise Guide

Building Self-Esteem

1 Identify your *bottom line* and create a new one.

2 Challenge *rules for living.*

3 Make a list of everything you are good at, or used to be good at, and make a point of reading it every day.

4 Make a daily list of tasks you want to accomplish, and review it every evening.

5 Ask close friends what is attractive about you. Write their comments down and read them daily.

6 Learn to identify negative thoughts, and stop them in their tracks. Don't focus on negative things, such as the state of your skin.

7 Learn to say no to people.

8 Reward yourself every day.

Reducing stress and anxiety

1 Don't multi-task.

2 Nurture your relationships.

3 Exercise at least three times a week for thirty minutes at a time. Shower afterwards.

4 Do the body scan daily.

5 Use the breathing technique used in the body scan any time you feel anxious or stressed.

6 Get enough sleep.

Lifestyle

1 Eat a balanced diet. Don't eat too much at one sitting. Limit your consumption of sugars and spicy food. Also, don't eat kelp.

2 Drink a lot of water. Limit your consumption of sweet drinks, alcohol and caffeine.

3 Take care in the sun.

4 Limit touching your skin.

5 Supplement. Take 30mg of zinc gluconate/glyconate and a 25 µg Vitamin D pill every day.

6 Cleanse. Try to shower twice a day. Use a gentle, non-comedogenic, cleanser.

7 Be careful about clothing and backpacks.

Appendix 2. The Product Method™-Concise Guide

Facial Acne Method Steps

How often?

For the first week, once a day, in the morning. After that, twice a day, once in the morning and once in the evening, ideally around twelve hours between applications.

1.   Cleanse

Wet your face, then, using your hands, wash it gently with the non-comedogenic cleanser for about ten seconds. *Do not use a cloth to wash*. Rinse with water until there is no cleanser left on your face. Dry gently with a soft towel, patting the towel on your face, *not* rubbing.

Wait about ten minutes for your skin to dry completely.

2.   Apply the 2.5% BP treatment

Firstly, wash and dry your hands well. For the first week use about ⅛ teaspoon/bean sized amount, a little more if you have acne on the front of your neck. After one week, gradually up the amount to about a teaspoon/grape sized amount (4ml) by the end of week 3.

Gently spread the BP around your face, avoiding the sensitive area around the eyes. *Do not rub the BP in.*

This should take no more than a minute or so. Wash and dry your hands.

Wait about ten minutes for the treatment to fully absorb into your skin.

3.   **Moisturise**

Wash and dry your hands. Use about a teaspoon/grape sized amount of non-comedogenic moisturiser, a little more if you also have acne on the front of your neck. Add sunscreen to the moisturiser if needed.

Gently spread the moisturiser around your face and neck. This should take no more than a minute, and will take about ten minutes to fully absorb. Wash and dry your hands.

Body/Neck Acne Method Steps

How often?

For the first week, once a day, in the morning. After that, twice a day, once in the morning and once in the evening, ideally around twelve hours between applications.

1.   **Cleanse**

This should be done in the shower. Firstly wet your face and body, then, using your hands, wash all acne prone areas gently with the non-comedogenic cleanser for no more than one minute in total. *Do not use a wash-cloth.* Rinse well until there is no cleanser left on your face or body. Dry gently with a soft towel, softly patting the towel on your face and body's acne prone areas, *not* rubbing.

Wait about ten minutes for your skin to dry completely.

2.   Apply the 2.5% BP treatment

Firstly wash and dry your hands well. If you get acne on the back and sides of the neck, use about a ½ teaspoon sized amount (2ml) of BP on these areas. For the chest and upper back/shoulders, use about a teaspoon/grape sized amount (4ml) for each side, which is a total of about 4 teaspoons. Use more if you get acne all the way down your back.

Gently spread the BP around the acne prone areas. *Do not rub the BP in.* This should take no more than two minutes to do. Wash and dry your hands.

Wait about ten minutes for the treatment to fully absorb into your skin.

3.   Apply the AHA

Firstly, wash and dry your hands well. If you get acne on the back and sides of the neck, use about a ½ teaspoon sized amount (2ml) of non-comedogenic AHA on these areas. For the chest and upper back/shoulders, use about a teaspoon sized amount (4ml) for each side, which is a total of about 4 teaspoons. Use more if you get acne all the way down your back. Add sunscreen to the AHA if needed.

Gently spread the AHA around the acne prone areas. *Do not rub the AHA in.* This should take no more than two minutes to do. Wash and dry your hands.

Wait a few minutes before putting on your shirt, in order to let the AHA fully absorb.

Appendix 3. Body Scan Transcript

Body Scan

Try to fit this meditation into your daily schedule. It should take about twenty minutes. The best time for me is late in the evening, but be aware that if you are tired, you may fall asleep! I find doing the meditation at home in my living room is best, but if you have a quiet private office that you want to use for example, then just switch off your phone and computer screen and that will be fine.

Sit down in your favourite chair. Loosen any tight clothing you might be wearing, for example a tie, belt or top button of a shirt. Make yourself comfortable.

Close your eyes and breathe in deeply through your nose, imagining you are inflating a balloon in your stomach. Count to 3 seconds and then breathe out through your nose for 3 seconds, deflating the balloon. Continue breathing in this way. If your mind becomes distracted, then focus again on your breathing.

After a minute or two, *continue with the deep breathing, but start to focus on your body*. Begin with your toes. Pay total attention in the moment as to how they feel. Are they hot or cold? Can you feel your socks or stockings against them? Describe the sensations in your mind in as much detail as you can.

Slowly work your way up your feet and then on to your calves and shins, describing everything to yourself. Carry on to your knees, your upper legs, and then to your groin and your buttocks. How does your behind feel against the chair? Hard? Soft? Cold? Warm?

Proceed to your lower back and then your middle back, describing any sensations you experience, for example the feeling against the chair. Then work your way across your shoulder blades and shoulder joints describing any textures or tension you feel.

Focus on your midriff and then your chest; perhaps you can feel the soft fabric of your T-shirt or blouse against your skin? Move to your fingers and then your hands, noticing the difference in temperature between the front of your hands and the back of your hands. Work your way up your arms, how do they feel against the arms of the chair? Does your skin feel warm beneath your shirt?

Then go up your neck, and on to your jaw and your mouth. Does your jaw feel relaxed, or is it tense? Are your lips tightly closed? Move up to your nose, can you feel the cool air when you breathe out? Proceed to your eyes. How do your eyelids feel? Relaxed? Focus on your forehead, and then your ears. Can you feel your hair brushing against them? Then work your way up to your scalp. Become fully aware of your whole body.

Continue with the deep breathing and consider which part of your body feels *most tense*. Focus on that part and try to visualise *which colour the tension feels like*.

Consider which part of your body feels *most relaxed*. What *colour does the relaxation feel like*?

As you breathe in, imagine you are breathing in the relaxing colour, filling your lungs with it and then transporting it around your body. Picture the colour healing your whole skin and body, filling it with calm relaxation.

As you breathe out, imagine you are expelling the colour of tension, like dragon smoke from your nostrils, taking all the stress and acne away.

Then totally focus on the positive colour as you breathe in and out. Imagine the positive colour relaxing your toes, slowly rising up your legs to your groin, relaxing your back and your shoulder blades, then your midriff, up your chest and into your fingers, bringing the colour up your arms to your neck, mouth, up to your forehead and, finally, your scalp and hair. Imagine your body full of the relaxed colour, relaxing every pore, muscle, tendon and organ.

Continue this for a short while then *think of a word* to describe your relaxed feeling. Focus on that word as you continue the deep breathing, letting it fill your body for a few minutes. Enjoy the feeling of being lost in total relaxation.

After a few minutes, slowly count backwards from five to one, gradually becoming more and more aware of your surroundings as you count. When you get to one, slowly open your eyes.

About The Author

I was born and brought up in bonnie Scotland, a land of mountains, lochs and hard drinking people. My educational and professional background is in environmental science. In my spare time, I like hiking in the mountains and reading good books. This is my first book.

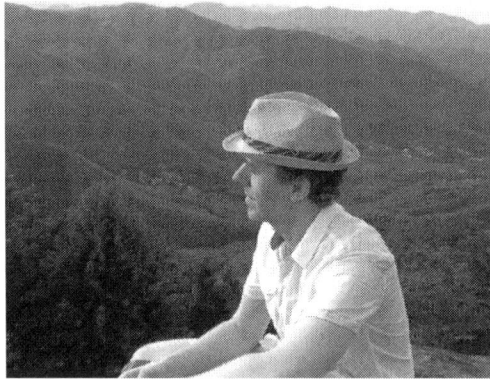

Andrew Duguid

March 2017

Thank you for reading this book.

Please review it on Amazon when you have time!

Printed in Great Britain
by Amazon

Management of Fire and Explosions

Conference Organizing Committee

P Bennett (Chair)
CSE International Limited

F Crawley
W S Atkins

G Dalzell
BP Exploration Operating Co Limited

G Essery
Society of Industrial Emergency Services
Officers

B Fullam
Health & Safety Executive

L Goldstone
The Institution of Electrical Engineers

R Hadwin
Royal & Sun Alliance

N Jones
University of Liverpool

I Lawrenson
Hazards Forum

R Mudge
Det Norske Veritas

T Pretious
Home Office

H Stone

Thanks also go to the Fire Safety Association.

IMechE
Conference Transactions

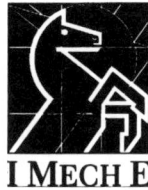

150th Anniversary

1847 - 1997

International Conference on

Management of Fire and Explosions

8–9 December 1997, IMechE, HQ, London, UK
28–29 April 1998, UMIST Conference Centre, Manchester, UK

Organized by the Environmental, Health and Safety Group of
the Institution of Mechanical Engineers (IMechE)
and the Hazards Forum

Sponsored by the Fire Protection Association

Co-sponsored by:
The Emergency Planning Society
The Health and Safety Executive
Society of Industrial Emergency Services Officers
The Royal Aeronautical Society
The Institution of Chemical Engineers
The Institution of Electrical Engineers
The Institution of Civil Engineers
Institute of Fire Safety

IMechE Conference Transaction 1997 – 5

Published by Mechanical Engineering Publications Limited for
the Institution of Mechanical Engineers, Bury St Edmunds and London.

© The Institution of Mechanical Engineers 1997

ISSN 1356–1448
ISBN 1 86058 101 3

A CIP catalogue record for this book is available from the British Library.

Printed by Antony Rowe Limited, Chippenham, Wilts. UK

Contents

Related Titles of Interest

For the full range of titles published by MEP contact:

Sales Department
Mechanical Engineering Publications Limited
Northgate Avenue
Bury St Edmunds
Suffolk
IP32 6BW
UK

Tel: 01284 763277
Fax: 01284 704006

C537/001/97

UK fire safety legislation – an overview

A R EVERTON PhD, AIFireE
Faculty of Law, University of Leicester, UK

SYNOPSIS

The purpose of this paper is to provide an overview of the basic principles of fire safety law in the United Kingdom. Taking a historical perspective, it outlines the Common Law origins, and then traces the legal system's statutory growth through the parallel developments of Building Control and control over premises once occupied. It notes the defects of the law, deals with the continuing flow of reform and proposals for reform, and considers the divers pressures (including in particular the needs of European conformity and of 'de-regulation') influencing the future direction which the law may take.

1. THE COMMON LAW ORIGINS

For centuries, the law has been involved with fire safety. Injury or loss which is consequent upon the spread of fire has long concerned the courts. For instance, there echo down the years from as far back as the fifteenth century the words of Markham J. in Beaulieu v Finglam (1), who explained that a man might be liable for any person entering his house with his leave or knowledge "... if he does any act ..... with a candle or aught else ..... whereby [his] neighbour's house is burnt." And two centuries later, in Tuberville v Stamp (2), we find the observation being made that "every man ..... is bound to keep his fire safely and securely by day and by night." As time went by, the judges developed a number of mechanisms by means of which civil liability for such damage might be imposed, and, if we look in the law of torts today, we see it provided for by actions in nuisance and negligence, and too, by the existence of an independent strand of potential liability for damage caused by fire.

2. STATUTORY BUILDING CONTROLS : A MAJOR CONTRIBUTION

To the oblique advancement of fire safety made by the law of tort, there became added, however, a more direct contribution to that cause. Such were their extent, Parliament found the need to respond to the social and economic problems wrought by fire. And, along with the growth of fire insurance, the eighteenth century witnessed a series of enactments which led to the well known Fires Prevention (Metropolis) Act 1774, and which provided the germs of modern fire precautions through Building Control.

In the nineteenth century, a heightening of interest in public health saw an interest in the importance of Building Control. Sanitation was addressed in addition to fire safety, and it was sought to achieve a transition from merely local to national legislation. For the law makers in this arena the aim was clear (if its fulfilment difficult) : it was to establish a legal structure able effectively to cope with the adverse living and working conditions which the industrial revolution had spawned. If, though, the key objective in this period was to create an effective system for the meeting of public need, fresh demands were to be made of the legislators in the twentieth century.

As the present century progressed, with the pace of life quickening, and with innovations in building techniques, the fashioners of Building Control were to face new and somewhat different aspirations. Without any loss of efficacy, the need was perceived for a régime which simultaneously provided flexibility.

In the furtherance of this aim, we in our time have seen a series of major, complex reforms. Through the early decades of this century, fire safety via Building Control relied on bye-laws which were made by local authorities to a centrally issued model. Eventually, this rather clumsy system gave way to nationally applicable "Building Regulations" (3) but, in due course, these too fell from favour on the grounds of undue intricacy and rigidity. And by the mid 1980s, in keeping with the de-regulatory spirit of the day, major reform emerged. Such was its extent, moreover, it was phased.

First, in 1985, came the recasting of the form of Building Control. The burdensome Building Regulations of 1976 (4) were replaced by a set of Building Regulations couched in broad functional terms (5) and supported by non-mandatory technical guidance in "Approved Documents". Then, in the next stage, content was addressed, and this culminated with the appearance of the Building Regulations, 1991 (6).

Of its very nature, the fire safety aspect of Building Control has always been at the heart of the reformers' thinking, and, reflecting the caution for which the subject calls, it has been only in gradual steps that the current pattern of fire related requirements has been brought about. Very briefly it may be explained thus:- All the fire safety components of the current Regulations (embracing internal and external fire spread, means of escape, and the facilitation of assistance to the fire service) are expressed - like other components - as general, functional requirements (7). They are supported by non-mandatory technical guidance, and they are made applicable to nearly all new and altered buildings.

The saga of the promotion of fire safety through Building Control is thus one of continuous progression. Developing both in sophistication and sphere of influence, it also provided the core for the addition of wider public health provisions, and remained central to a blossoming régime.

3. IMPORTANT PARALLEL CONTROL, i.e. OVER OCCUPIED PREMISES

In the field of fire safety law the Building Control saga tells only half the story. This is because its control extends only over new and altered buildings. The legal regulation of fire safety in premises once occupied has its own distinct system, and moreover an intricate history. To this second aspect of the overall picture we now have to turn.

By way of introduction it may be observed that whereas this other branch of fire safety law shares the aspiration of the fire component of Building Control, its articulation is less coherent. On account of the way in which it has grown, it is a fragmented system - fragmented in its substantive provisions, its enforcement techniques and its enforcing agencies. Rooted in efforts to deal with the problematic consequences of industrialisation, the relevant legal provisions were to grow in 'piecemeal' fashion. Not only that, they slowly came to embrace an enormous range of widely differing types of premises (8).

The 'patchwork' like character of the régime led naturally to increasing criticism, which, in its turn, fostered demands for rationalisation. Partly in consequence of this, the latter half of this century has been a period of reformatory zeal. The reform pathway has proved (indeed still proves) far from an easy one, its route marked by a succession of endeavours, achievements and yet further endeavours.

The initial step of major importance was the enactment of the Fire Precautions Act, 1971, the first Act to be exclusively devoted to the subject. It established a control framework based on the designation and compulsory certification of premises posing risk to human life. Then, not long after, with a view to subjecting general fire precautions in public and industrial premises to the same regulatory structure, its ambit was extended by the Health and Safety at Work Act, 1974 to cover places of work. Under the umbrella of these statutes, and over the next few years, numerous industrial and commercial premises were subjected to the control system, and thus a considerable degree of rationalisation was achieved. Even so, however, the defect of fragmentation was not overcome, and for a simple reason. While it had been intended that the certification régime of the 1971 Act should be used to render obsolete much of the pre-existing scattered provision, cost proved an insurmountable obstacle.

With early hopes thus unfulfilled, this branch of fire law was to proceed even to the present day characterised by fragmentation. At its centre would be the Fire Precautions Act, with numerous other specific provisions making their own particular contribution to the scene (9).

The scale of the '70s reforms were not to be matched in the '80s, vibrant though the decade was. From an increasing urge to return responsibility to the individual came a call for the ending of fire certification, but so great a change remained elusive. Nevertheless, the need for a more flexible approach was plain, and measures, albeit modest, were taken to this end. While certification was retained, Part One of the Fire Safety and Safety of Places of Sport Act, 1987 so modified the structure as, inter alia, to confine more closely the coverage of the certification process (10).

4. FIRE SAFETY IN THE '90s, THE ZEAL FOR REFORM UNABATING

In spite of the move mentioned above, the onerous qualities of the Fire Precautions Act were not assuaged, and for this reason amongst others it was destined to stay in the sights of the law reformers. As we moved into the '90s, and as the early years of the current decade progressed, so the Act was to be the focus of considerable reformatory enthusiasm - enthusiasm, furthermore, which has not waned.

The present author has observed elsewhere (11) that the spirit for legal change has been marked by "... a succession of explorations, appraisals (12) and European conformity efforts" (13). It has been noted that the whole endeavour has been influenced by pressure including both needs and desiderata. The needs, it was explained, were to "... ensure compliance with EC law, to rationalise the law, and to overcome enforcement problems at the interface between control over new and altered premises and over premises once occupied" (14). The desiderata, it was explained, embraced "the search for de-regulation, the urge to modernise the law so as to move from prescription to 'goal based' duties, to give prominence to risk assessment, and to accommodate innovation" (15).

A milestone of particular significance was reached in May 1996 when the then Home Office Minister announced a series of proposals designed to rationalise and simplify the system, to keep safety standards high, and, at the same time, to lighten the burden borne by business. Amongst them were proposals to give fire authorities greater scope to exempt from certification 'non high risk' premises, to target certification more accurately at 'high risk premises', and to clarify the respective responsibilities of Building Control and fire authorities in the arena of new buildings.

Since the making of the announcement, there has been the General Election and a change of administration. It is believed though, that the needs which those proposals sought to meet remain unaffected, and that the question continues as to how and when they might be met. This, though, is an issue for the longer term. At the time of writing, the most prominent matter is the implementation of the fire safety components of the EC Framework and Workplace Directives (16). The Regulations which implement these components, namely the Fire Precautions (Workplace) Regulations 1997 (17), are at present the cynosure of the fire community, and we have now to consider them.

5. FOCUS ON THE WORKPLACE REGULATIONS

To begin with, certain observations are in point by way of background. The Regulations were laid before Parliament on July 29th 1997, and should come into effect on December 1st 1997. Their emergence, in what promises to be their final form, follows a long and difficult period of gestation in which the tension between the legal obligation to implement the EC Directives' requirements and grave fears of over burdening business, resulted in a series of revisions and withdrawals.

At the time of their being signed, the Home Office issued a news release in which reference was made to these troubling circumstances, (a reference which testified to the continuance by the current administration of the 'de-regulatory' climate so carefully fostered by its predecessor). It was intimated in the release that the revised Regulations had as their objectives the advancement of the existing high standards of fire safety, and of so doing at minimal cost to business, - the latter aim being possible, it was noted, because of the generally sound level of fire safety which was already provided.

On the same day, Mr. Howarth, The Parliamentary Under-Secretary of State, also emphasised (18) the 'minimalistic' quality of the Regulations. They were written, he advised, in 'copy out' language so as to ensure an effectual but not an 'over' implementation of the Directives' requirements, and further, their enforcement régime imported safeguarding procedures from the De-Regulation and Contracting Out Act, 1994 in order to ensure that in this context business was handled with 'a light touch'.

On account of the combination of aspirations which they had to meet, and because they had both to add to, and blend with, an already complex legal picture (19), it is scarcely surprising that they should be elaborate. Accordingly, that which now follows can be no more than an outline of their basic thrust.

Extending to Great Britain, the purpose of the Regulations is to make provision for minimum fire standards in places where people work. To this end, Part II contains a number of specific requirements with which every employer has to comply in respect of workplaces, other than excepted workplaces, which are under his control (20). Regulation 3 contains a lengthy list of excepted premises which are closely controlled in other ways (21), and at the heart of which are workplaces comprising fire certificated premises (though not including premises with a 'deemed' certificate) (22).

The specific requirements are set out in Regulations 4, 5 and 6. Regulation 4 imposes requirements relating to the equipping of workplaces with appropriate fire-fighting equipment, fire detectors and alarms. It obliges employers to take fire fighting measures (23), nominate workers to implement them, and arrange fire brigade contacts. Regulation 5 addresses itself to the ensuring of the state, nature, adequacy and indication of emergency routes and exits. And Regulation 6 is concerned to ensure the technical maintenance of the workplace, and of the equipment and devices to which Regulations 4 and 5 relate.

While the requirements appear at first sight extensive, the manner in which they are framed emphasises the circumscribed base from which they proceed. The Regulations make it plain that their requirements impinge only "where necessary" and "in order to safeguard the safety of employees in case of fire." Again, Regulation 4 demands only the equipping of a workplace "... to the extent that it is appropriate", what is "appropriate" to be determined by matters including the dimensions, use and contents of the building.

Before moving on, one further point must be made on Part II. Regulation 3(1) obliges an employer to comply with its requirements in respect of every workplace "... which is to any extent under his control." What of any parts over which he does not have control? This issue is met by Regulation 3(2), which places a responsibility on persons who do have that control to ensure compliance (24).

In contrast with the specific precautionary matters embraced by Part II of the Regulations, Part III deals with general requirements. Under its provisions, an employer is obliged, inter alia, to carry out a fire risk assessment to identify necessary measures to comply with the specific requirements, to organise those measures effectively, to give employees fire related information and to ensure the co-ordination of fire safety measures in shared buildings.

The implementation of the EC's general requirements into the domestic law of the UK is neatly executed. Part III achieves its purpose by amending where necessary the relevant regulations of the Management of Health and Safety at Work Regulations, 1992 (25). By way of a leading illustration of the approach, we may instance the pivotal obligations involving the making of a fire risk assessment. Regulation 3 of the 1992 Regulations which, in its original form, casts a duty on employers to make a risk assessment for the identification of measures necessary to comply with health and safety provisions, is amended by Regulation 8 of the Regulations now under discussion so as expressly to oblige him also to take such action in the area of fire risk (26). To extend the law in this way is elegant, though perhaps confusing for the non-lawyer.

At this point, we may turn from substance to enforcement. This is the burden of Part IV of the Regulations, which casts the duty of enforcement on the fire authorities (27). Striving, as earlier noted, for a 'lightness of touch', Part IV puts forward a 'graded system', distinguishing between 'serious' and 'other than serious' cases, and dealing with them separately.

First there are addressed the 'serious cases'. Regulation 11 renders guilty of an offence a person who intentionally or negligently fails to comply with any provision of the workplace fire precautions legislation where the failure places employees at serious risk in case of fire. And, for this purpose, 'at serious risk' means being subjected to a risk of death or serious injury which is likely to materialise.

Continuing the theme of 'serious cases', a fire authority may, under Regulation 13, serve an 'enforcement notice' on a person where they are of the opinion that there has been a failure to comply with the provisions and in consequence employees have been placed at 'serious risk'. Putting in place an elaborate system for the safeguarding of business, the notice must state why the opinion is held, specify remedial steps, require them to be taken in a specified term, and advert to the appeals procedure. Further, unless the risk is too serious for delay, the fire authority must first give a notice stating that they are proposing to serve a notice, their reasons and its terms, and give opportunity for representations (28).

A right of appeal to the magistrates' court from an enforcement notice is conferred on a person by Regulation 14. And a most important point to note in this connection is that the bringing of an appeal does not have the effect of suspending the operation of the notice unless the court so directs (29). The subject of enforcement notices is then completed by Regulation 15, which makes it an offence to contravene the requirements of such a notice.

Thence, the Regulations turn their attention to 'other than serious cases'. Under Regulation 16, in situations of a failure to comply with the Regulations' requirements which do not warrant the issuing of an enforcement notice, the fire authority can apply to the County Court for an 'enforcement order'. If the Court is satisfied that the person in question is obliged to take action to comply with the requirements, it can order him so to act. Again, before making any such application to the Court, the fire authority must give the person against whom they propose to proceed a notice intimating their proposal, their reasons and necessary remedial steps, and must afford opportunity for representations (30).

From even so short a sketch of the enforcement provisions, the keenness of the desire to be 'business friendly' is plain. The extent of the reliance on civil law is notable, resort being had to criminal sanctions only in the very limited arena where the failure to comply with the requirements places employees at 'serious risk'. And not only that, the protective procedures established by the Regulations means that even in the case of the more common (i.e. 'other than serious') situation, the actual use of civil proceedings will be very much a last resort. As the Home Office News Release of 29th July 1997 explains, much effort has gone into devising a means of giving "... fire authorities and businesses the opportunity to discuss and remedy any minor breaches and failures rather that resort to the courts ..."

How this new approach of a 'risk appropriate' régime will work in practice, and how effective it proves in fire safety terms is, of course, something which remains to be seen. Naturally, it is a matter of striking a balance, and in the arena of fire safety, where the likelihood and consequences of risk may be quite disproportionate, to strike it successfully has always been of the utmost difficulty.

For a number of reasons it has been thought fit to dwell on these new Regulations. Long awaited, they have inevitably taken the limelight. They have at their heart the fashionable concept of risk assessment, and they place responsibility for fire safety fairly and squarely on the individual. Moreover, by importing safeguards from the De-regulation and Contracting Out Act, 1994, they seek to establish an enforcement system characterised by 'lightness of touch'.

6. THE FUTURE : 'ROOT AND BRANCH' REFORM?

In spite of the current attention paid to these Regulations, their significance must not be over-emphasised. They only constitute a further (albeit vivid) patch in the patchwork quilt of laws governing fire precautions in premises already occupied (31). Far more significant would be a 'root and branch' reform of this colourful legal scenario ~ and to that issue we must briefly turn by way of conclusion.

Any fundamental reform of the area of law dealing with fire precautions in premises once occupied cannot be other than a fraught venture. Amongst the many attendant difficulties there may be included for consideration the following facts:-

a) That the scattered enactments of which the law is comprised are so numerous, and, having been produced at different times, reflect different philosophies of approach.

b) That the fragmented character of the law is a fragmentation not only of substance but also of enforcement 'tools' and agencies.

c) That the Fire Precautions Act's certification system which lies at the heart of the matter is widely regarded as being - to the extent of its present coverage - unduly burdensome and costly.

d) That in many situations fire safety requirements cannot be completely separated from other relevant requirements (32).

e) That because it has long been thought best to separate fire law into two main branches, with controls in premises once occupied dealt with independently of those in new and altered premises, there is the problem (by no means at present overcome) of ensuring the seamless interlocking of the two régimes.

f) That the law now has to accommodate requirements emanating from European directives.

From this list there emerge certain aspirations for a new law to meet. It can be contended that its prime objectives should, perhaps, be these:-

First, to rationalise the existing law and so to render coherent that which is currently so "piecemeal".

Secondly, to dovetail the law relating to premises once occupied with Building Control in such a way as to achieve a 'seamless' flow.

Thirdly, to solve the problem as to the appropriate scope and extent of the 'certification' process.

Fourthly, to accommodate without strain any European requirements.

The matter does not, however, rest there. Current policy and philosophy pose further desiderata. Received wisdom appears to expect that new law should be flexible, and, too, impose no burdens further than those which are appropriate. Again, it should be 'goal based' rather than overly prescriptive. Other features deemed laudable include the placing of responsibility on the individual, and the ensuring of 'self compliance'. Yet again, at its core must be the fashionable notion of 'risk assessment'. And yet again, enforcement has to be 'risk appropriate', and the tools and techniques of enforcement 'user friendly'.

Indeed, the law reformers seem to be obliged to meet so many needs that they face a particularly daunting task. With the appearance in early 1997 of the Fire Brigade Union's Fire Safety Bill, a considerable reformatory endeavour was launched, but while in the event it did not progress, it showed the taking on board of much current thinking in the search for advancement.

Clearly, there is still a long way to go. And, while the journey is in the process of being made, it could be asked whether thought might be given to the eventual scope of the public

C537/001 © IMechE 1997

law of fire safety. Historically, it has been concerned with the saving of life, but why should it not enjoy a wider remit? In addition to the protection of life, why should it not embrace the protection of property, or even, in an age when 'green' issues prove a continuing focus, the protection of the environment? Fire itself does not differentiate. So, perhaps, even with hesitance, we could ask 'why should the law?'.

REFERENCES

1.   (1401) YB Pasch. 2 Hen. 4f. 18 pl. 6.
2.   (1697) 3 Ld. Raym. 375.
3.   See the Public Health Act, 1961, Section 4. The Regulations were applicable throughout most of England and Wales; (London occupied a special position).
4.   S.I. 1976/1676.
5.   S.I. 1985/1065.
6.   S.I. 1991/2768.
7.   See Schedule 1 to the Regulations Part B 1-5.
8.   - including, for instance, places of work (such as offices, shops and factories), and places where people resort in numbers, such as places of entertainment, premises selling intoxicants, gaming establishments, and institutions like schools and residential homes.
9.   In Annex F to "Fire Safety Legislation & Enforcement" (The Report of the Interdepartmental Review Team, DTI, 1994) there are listed some fifty pieces of primary legislation with fire safety provisions. Taking simply random instances of the contributory strands, housing legislation addresses houses in multiple occupation, schools and 'social care' legislation deals with various residential institutions, and theatre, cinemas and music and dancing legislation attends to places of entertainment.
10. The régime established by the 1971 Act produced 'overkill' in that, because it worked on numerical cut-off, it subjected to the certification process too many 'low risk' premises. The 1987 Act sought to render the system less burdensome by adding a further discretionary escape route for certain 'low risk' premises from the need for a certificate. (But exemption, from the need for a certificate, by whatever route, does not mean 'low risk' premises are uncontrolled. They are still caught by basic requirements, which indeed are set to become more elaborate).
11   "Fire Prevention", 294 November 1996 p.16.
12   - including for instance the Home Office Review of the Fire Precautions Act in 1993 and the Report of the Interdepartmental Review Team on Fire Safety Legislation and Enforcement in 1994.
13. - efforts relating to the problematic implementation of the fire safety elements of certain EC Health and Safety Directives (as to which more follows shortly).
14. See footnote 11 above.
15. Ibid.
16. 89/331 EEC and 89/654 EEC respectively. (these Directives were brought in to encourage the enhancement of workers' health and safety, and to set minimum health and safety requirements for the great majority of work places).
17. S.I. 1997 No. 1840.
18. - by means of a 'written answer'.

19. The requirement of the EC Directives which these Regulations are designed to meet are founded purely in "worker protection", but the fire safety for workers in the UK is part of an intricate legal scene in which that aim mingles with others, and is pursued by different statutes in different ways. In order to fit into the already existing, relevant parts of the domestic law the Regulations are so made as simultaneously to 'belong' to fire safety law, yet to 'partake of the character' of health and safety at work law.

20. Reg. 3(1).

21. - including underground railways and 'special' premises under, respectively, the Fire Precautions (Sub-surface Railway Stations) Regulations 1989, (S.I. 1989 No. 1401 as amended) and the Fire Certificates (Special Premises) Regulations 1976, (S.I. 1976 No. 2003).

22. - 'deemed' under Sched. 8 para. 2 to the Health and Safety at Work Act, 1974 (i.e. old means of escape certificates issued under the Factories Act, 1961 and the Offices, Shops and Railway Premises Act, 1963). Note too, and importantly, that workplaces covered by licensing legislation are not included in the list of excepted premises.

23. - such as the creation of an emergency plan of action.

24. Such a person will usually be the owner or landlord.

25. S.I. 1992 No. 2051.

26. It is envisaged that fire risk assessments may be carried out as part of the general health and safety risk assessment, or as a separate exercise.

27. See Regulation 10.

28. The fire authority must consider any representations which are duly made; (Regulation 13(3)(c)).

29. - upon an application made by the appellant.

30. Once more, the fire authority must consider any representations; (Regulation 16(2)(c)).

31. A further step along the reform path, though its mission is as yet only inchoate, was the emergence in 1996 of a Consultation Paper on the widening of exemption from the certification process under the Fire Precautions Act, 1971 (as amended).

32. While the health and safety of persons at work is a prime illustration of the point, another may be found in the protection of the theatre going public, (see the Theatres Act, 1968 Section 12(1) and Schedule 1).

C537/001 © IMechE 1997

C537/003/97

The scope and scale of the United Kingdom's fire problem

W DAILEY PhD, CChem, FRSC
The Loss Prevention Council, Borehamwood, UK

SYNOPSIS

This paper presents an overall view of the scope and the scale of the fire problem in the United Kingdom over the period 1986 to 1995. It presents data on such matters as the number of fires per year, the annual toll of fire deaths and injuries, the principal causes of fire deaths, annual fire losses, the principal causes of fires, and the occupancies suffering the highest fire losses. The paper also makes brief reference to some of the more significant fires that have occurred during, or near to, the period under consideration.

1 THE EFFECTS OF FIRES

The principal effects of fires are life loss and injury, financial losses, job losses, loss of our heritage - the destruction by fire of historic buildings and their contents, environmental damage, and, for businesses, the loss of profits that may result from the interruption of business activity that so often follows a fire.

The fires at Bradford City Football Club in 1985(56 deaths), at King's Cross underground station in 1987(31 deaths), on the Piper Alpha oil rig in 1988(165 deaths), and at the London cinema club in 1994(11 deaths) are but examples of recent fires that have caused multiple deaths.

The fires at Ministry of Defence warehousing in Donnington in 1983 and 1988 resulted in estimated losses of £164m and £184m respectively and, in the case of the second fire, the release of large quantities of asbestos dust into the atmosphere constituted a pollution of the environment.

Fires at Hampton Court Palace in 1986, Uppark House in 1989, and Windsor Castle in 1992 are well known examples of fires in historic buildings that resulted in losses to our cultural heritage.

A fire at a Nottinghamshire printing works in the summer of 1996 provided a very recent example of financial loss arising from the interruption of business activity. The insured loss covering the material damage caused by the fire was £11.25m, and the losses suffered as a result of business interruption were estimated to be £10m.

2 NUMBERS OF FIRE DEATHS AND INJURIES

Fire deaths and injuries in the United Kingdom over the period 1986 to 1995 are shown in table 1 (1).

Table 1

Year	Number of Deaths	Number of Injuries
1986	957	12768
1987	929	12567
1988	915	13376
1989	901	14159
1990	898	14041
1991	816	14714
1992	807	14720
1993	720	14625
1994	699	16866
1995	808	17234

Given that approximately 75% of fire deaths occur in the home, the steady fall in the annual death toll from 1986 to 1994, with the 1994 figure being the lowest since 1962, was almost certainly due to the success of campaigns to encourage people to fit smoke alarms in their homes; currently some 75% of dwellings are fitted with smoke alarms.

The number of fatalities recorded for 1994 and 1995 include those that occurred in two additional categories of incidents - "late fire calls " and "heat and smoke damage only" - that were not previously categorized as fires.

The number of injuries has continued to rise, the figure for 1995 being the highest ever recorded. This rise may be apparent rather than real in that whilst, in years gone by, someone who had inhaled a lungful of smoke would have been taken in by a neighbour and given a cup of tea, today the tendency is to refer them for a precautionary medical check-up thereby turning them into an "injury" statistic.

3 CAUSES OF FIRE DEATHS

The numbers of fire deaths from various causes, expressed as a percentage of the total number of fire deaths, in the United Kingdom in 1995 are shown in table 2 (1).

Table 2

Cause of death	Percentage of deaths
Overcome by smoke or gas	37%
Burns	26%
Burns and overcome by smoke or gas	18%
Other	6%
Unspecified	13%

The figures for 1995 are, in general, in agreement with those for the other years in the period under review. Clearly, the biggest single cause of death is inhalation of the smoke and gas produced by the fire. These consists of a mixture of particulate matter and a lethal cocktail of chemicals that commonly includes such substances as ammonia, carbon monoxide, ethanoic acid, hydrogen chloride, hydrogen cyanide, hydrogen sulphide, and oxides of both nitrogen and sulphur.

4 THE NUMBERS OF FIRES

The numbers of fires per year, from 1986 to 1995 are shown in table 3 (1).

Table 3

Year	Number of fires (Thousands)
1986	387
1987	354
1988	356
1989	456
1990	467
1991	436
1992	426
1993	451
1994	479
1995	604

Two points are worthy of note in connection with the numbers of fires. First, the number of fires in 1995 was the highest ever recorded. Most of this large (26%) increase in the number of fires may be attributed to an increase in the number of outdoor (grassland and heathland) fires, which no doubt were a direct result of the fact that we experienced a long, hot, summer in 1995.

Secondly, and of more concern than the record number of fires in 1995, is the general increase in the number of fires per year that began in 1989. Up until then, with the exceptions of 1976 and 1984 - when the hot summers resulted in many more outdoor (grassland and heathland) fires - the numbers of fires per year had, since 1969, remained fairly constant at some three hundred thousand. It is of some interest that the dramatic increase of one hundred thousand that occurred in 1989 coincided with what was probably the peak of the financial recession. A possible explanation of this increase will be given under fire losses.

5 THE DISTRIBUTION OF FIRES

For the period under review, the total numbers of fires, and the numbers occurring in various locations, are shown in table 4 (1). The figures are the numbers of fires, in thousands.

Table 4

Year	Total Number of fires	Number in dwellings	Number in other buildings	Number of outdoor fires	Number of chimney & other* fires
1986	387	64	42	228	54
1987	354	63	41	201	49
1988	356	64	42	209	41
1989	456	65	46	309	37
1990	467	63	45	326	33
1991	436	64	43	290	39
1992	426	65	43	283	35
1993	451	65	43	308	35
1994	479	64	45	338	34
1995	604	65	46	461	32

* the other fires in the last column of table 4 are "late call" and "heat and smoke damage only" fires that have been included only since 1984

The significant point that emerges from the figures in table 4 is that regardless of the total number of fires, or the numbers occurring elsewhere, the numbers of fires in buildings remains remarkably constant at close to one hundred thousand fires per year; with an almost constant 60%, 40% split between fires in dwellings and fires in other buildings

6 THE CAUSES OF FIRES

In this section, the cause of a fire is to be understood as the source of ignition. The statistics of the principal causes of fires differ somewhat depending upon whether one is looking at all fires in buildings, or solely at "Large" fires in buildings. A large fire is defined by the Fire Protection Association as one that resulted in losses that were equal or greater than £50,000. Although large fires do sometimes occur in places other than buildings, the overwhelming majority do occur in buildings.

6.1 The causes of all fires in buildings

In 1995, 31% of all fires in buildings were started deliberately, and in 2% of the cases the cause was either unknown or was under investigation. The remaining 67% of fires started accidentally and, for these accidental fires, the percentages resulting from various causes are shown in table 5 (1).

Table 5

Cause	Percentage of fires
Cooking appliances	37%
Electrical faults/misuse	18%
Smoking and matches	12%
Blowlamps, welding, and cutting	3%
Other	30%

The reason why cooking appliances are the largest single cause of these accidental fires is that there were approximately twice as many accidental fires in dwellings as there were in other buildings. Whilst dwellings will almost invariably be equipped with cookers, this is far less likely to be the case non-dwelling premises. Electrical causes should be understood as faults in, or misuse of, both electrical appliances and electrical distribution systems - wiring and flexes. As a cause of fire, "Smoking and matches" means the careless disposal of smoking materials and/or matches. Fires resulting from the use of blowlamps, or welding or cutting equipment, are, in many cases, caused by the activities of contractors. The £6.9m fire at Uppark House in 1989 was caused by roofing contractors using an oxy-acetylene welding torch.

6.2 The causes of large fires

At the time of writing, the Fire Protection Association's Large Fire Analysis for 1995 had not been published and therefore the data relating to the causes of large fires has been taken from the Association's Large Fire Analysis for 1994 (2). In that year there were 509 large fires in the United Kingdom , all of which occurred in buildings, and of which 46% were started deliberately or possibly deliberately, in 9% of the cases the cause was either under unknown or under investigation, and the remaining 45% were started accidentally. The causes of the accidentally started large fires in 1994 are shown in Table 6.

Table 6

Cause	Percentage of fires
Electrical faults/misuse	52%
Smoking and matches	14%
Blowlamps, welding, cutting, & use of fuels	7%
Gas appliances	6%
Unspecified appliances	3%
Other	18%

As has already been noted, some 60% of all of the fires in buildings occurred in dwellings, whilst none of the large fires did, and therefore the data in tables 5 and 6 allow some general comparisons to be made between the causes of fire - both deliberate and accidental - in domestic and workplace premises.

First, the incidence of deliberately set fires - arson - is some 50% higher in the workplace. Secondly, for accidental fires in the workplace, electrically caused fires are almost three times as likely, fires caused by smoking are equally likely, and contractors are twice as likely to start a fire.

7 FIRE LOSSES

7.1 Losses for all fires

The total estimated insured fire losses, for all fires, in the period under review are shown in table 7 (3).

Table 7

Year	Loss in £m
1986	456
1987	638
1988	646
1989	792
1990	1007
1991	1019
1992	850
1993	646
1994	615
1995	701

As can be seen, there was a rapid escalation of the losses in the second half of the eighties culminating with losses in excess of one billion pounds in both 1990 and 1991. At what was probably the height of the financial recession we were, on average, sending up in smoke and flames almost three million pounds worth of our industrial and commercial base every day of the year. The fact that the losses peaked at the height of the recession was, almost certainly, not simply an unrelated coincidence. Arson is believed to be the most common large insurance fraud and, with businesses in financial difficulties, it was hardly surprising that losses reached record levels. Support for this explanation of the increase in losses is to be found in a speech given by David McIntosh, a leading insurance lawyer, at the Chartered Institute of Loss Adjusters in 1990. He is reported (4) as having said that "the recession is expected to prompt respectable executives to consider arson and fraud rather than face the bankruptcy courts".

7.2 Cumulative losses for large fires

Table 8 shows the occupancies that sustained the largest cumulative losses from large fires in the period 1990 to 1994 (2).

Table 8

Occupancy	Cumulative loss in £m
Education	166
Insurance, banking, & business services	149
Retail distribution	134
Dwellings	109
Recreational & cultural services	74
Wholesale distribution	68
Food drink & tobacco	64

Educational establishments head the list because of the very large number of fires - especially in schools, which are a favourite target for the arsonist - rather than because of a few very costly fires. The figure for dwellings is abnormally high because it includes the costs of the fire at Windsor Castle in 1992 (£40m). Similarly, the figure for insurance, banking & business services has been greatly inflated by the cost of just one fire - that at the London Underwriting Centre in 1991. This fire alone cost £105m , and this sum does not include the figure for consequential loss.

8 DISTRIBUTION OF ARSON ATTACKS

It has already been noted that arson is the largest single cause of large fires. Arson is without doubt the most worrying aspect of the United Kingdom's fire problem, and it is one that is getting worse rather than better. It is therefore of interest to see where the arsonist is most likely to strike. In 1995 there were 250 large fires that were started deliberately. The percentage of these attacks suffered by various occupancies is shown in table 9 (5).

Table 9

Occupancy	Percentage of attacks
Industry	23%
Education	14%
Unoccupied buildings	11%
Dwellings	8%
Shops	4%
Warehouses	4%
Pubs, hotels, restaurants	4%
Agriculture	1%
Offices	1%
Other	30%

9 CONCLUSION

The purpose of this paper was to present such a selection of data as to give an overall picture of the nature and scale of the fire problem in the United Kingdom. Without such information it is difficult for the non-specialist to appreciate just how serious the problem is, and unless we understand the nature of the problem we can't even begin to tackle it. Its most worrying aspect is, of course, the loss of life and the often horrific injuries that result from fires but, as I hope has been demonstrated, fire also poses a very real threat to the health of our national economy. In the view of this writer, fire is the most serious single threat facing any business enterprise.

If we are to reduce, or even contain, the problem, those who are responsible for our industrial and commercial enterprises, those who run our health and education services, and those who are custodians of our cultural heritage, must surely give a much greater priority, and allocate the necessary resources, to training in the management of fire safety. .

10 REFERENCES

1. Summary Fire Statistics United kingdom 1995, published by the Home Office.
2. Fire Prevention, Vol. 299, May 1997, pp38-45.
3. Fire Prevention ,Vol. 294, November 1996, p31.
4. The Guardian, 6th September 1990.
5. Fire Prevention, Vol. 298, April 1997, p36.

Fire Prevention is the journal of the Fire Protection Association, which is a component part of the Loss Prevention Council.

C537/004/97

Design

M A WILLIAMS BSc, MICE, MIHT, MIOSH
Health and Safety Consultant

SYNOPSIS

The construction industry has a very poor accident record and traditional contracts separated the functions of client, designer and contractor. Designers concentrated on the performance of completed projects, which often led to design becoming important factors in construction accidents, as discussed. Designers should therefore possess expertise in the practicalities of construction to improve the safety and constructability of their work and the CDM Regulations have formalised this process, improving the industry's safety culture by placing responsibilities for the construction process on all the parties to contracts, including clients.

THE BACKGROUND - CONSTRUCTION INDUSTRY SAFETY

In dealing with design and its relationship to a safety culture, construction engineering will be used as an analogue and a basis for discussion due to its wide distribution and essential contribution to almost all industrial activity and in this context, construction is taken as including civil and structural engineering, together with building operations and demolition, all of which call for the participation of a very broad range of professions and trades. Almost invariably, no industry can exist without preliminary and continuing construction work and it is also unfortunately the case that many accidents in other industries have been caused by construction work or related operations.

The construction industry itself has a poor safety record and statistics show that over a very long period it has been one of the major sources of fatal and other accidents, not only to its own work force, but also the public at large. While most industrial processes are contained within factory buildings or secure site boundaries, construction is everywhere and all of us are often likely to be near or even passing through a construction site, hence increasing the risk of involvement if or when an incident occurs. This is borne out by figures published recently by the Health and Safety Executive for the five-year period from 1991/92 to 1995/96, for which the numbers of fatal injuries and corresponding fatal injury rates for construction work and the manufacturing industries, were as follows:

	Construction		Manufacturing	
	Number	Injury Rate*	Number	Injury Rate*
Employees	348	7.9	264	1.4
Self-employed	102	2.7	22	1.7
Public	25	-	4	-
Totals	475		290	

(* Rate per 100,000 workers)

Source: Health and Safety Commission – Annual Report 1995/96 (1)

The disproportionate numbers of fatalities caused by construction is further emphasised by the fatal injury rates, which show a severity ratio of some 5:1 for fatalities to construction employees as against those working in factories. No study of accident figures like these should overlook the fact that beyond the personal injuries and fatalities, there are also the indirect effects on individuals, companies and the national economy that are not always fully taken into account, but which nonetheless cause serious losses of time, money and materials.

THE CONSTRUCTION INDUSTRY – RESPONSIBILITY FOR SAFETY

It is suggested that in the past the manner in which the construction industry was organised and managed, together with its contractual arrangements, led to the creation and maintenance of a framework of 'separation and demarcation' by those involved which may have been an important contributory factor in the high accident levels experienced in construction for a considerable number of years and which only now are showing a downward trend. Until comparatively recently, the common procedure for construction of a project by contract involved three main parties - client, consultant and contractor - where design of the permanent works would be the sole responsibility of the consultant or other specialist and distinctly separate areas of responsibility and involvement were maintained by the participants. Clients and consultants had virtually no duties under criminal law for safety or failures during the construction phase and as generally there was no contract between contractors and designers, the interests of the latter tended to be limited to dimensional accuracy, quality of materials and finishes, compliance with specifications and the satisfactory performance of the completed structure or project. For their part, having first selected a consultant, discussed their needs and provided the necessary finance, clients then frequently distanced themselves from projects. Furthermore, contractual arrangements, usually based on documents drafted by professional organisations and negotiated for clients by their consultants, emphasised the total responsibility of contractors for all aspects of the construction work.

In addition to their onerous contractual obligations, contractors were made responsible under Statutory Acts and Regulations for site safety, including temporary works and the stability and viability of structures designed by others, at all stages prior to completion. Building would be to a design which was directed solely toward safe performance of the finished structure, often with little consideration being given by the designer to problems of 'buildability', strength or stability which might arise during the construction phase and there have been many collapses and serious accidents which can be directly attributed to a failure on the part of designers either to recognise difficulties or to pass on information connected with potential dangers to health or safety during construction.

The contractual arrangements described above are common in the construction industry and, when coupled with legal requirements for safety resting largely on contractors, they probably occasioned, perhaps even encouraged, a form of isolationism on the part of designers. This could have resulted in attitudes and procedures which were not conducive to developing a 'safety culture' - if that is taken to be the adoption of a constructive attitude to safety which links, involves and depends on all those concerned with a project from beginning to end and accepts that work during the construction phase and feasibility of erection methods are an important part of a designer's responsibility.

It could well be that due to the demarcation boundaries established by the contract system described above, some designers have lacked sufficient experience of the practicalities of construction work and therefore were not competent to understand the problems which would arise when their design was assembled or built under site conditions, with all the vagaries of weather, work force skills and availability of plant and equipment. In addition to the creation of risk, many examples have been encountered where considerable difficulty has been experienced in constructing designs because of their complexity, inaccessibility or unsuitability, all of which have increased the cost and time involved and it should not be forgotten that while not always causing accidents, these are another form of loss directly attributable to design.

DESIGN AS A FACTOR IN FAILURES

For the purposes of this paper, when discussing design as a cause of or factor in failures, the construction phase of projects is considered particularly relevant as it this stage that involves active input and involvement by more than one party to the contract and experience has shown that this is when most design-related failures occur.

Incidents range widely in size and seriousness but seem to display common features which include, among others:

- inadequate ground investigations and site surveys
- no allowance for uncovenanted exterior influences
- lack of understanding of construction loadings
- materials or components differing from specification
- changes of design without reference to original designer
- use of inappropriate standard designs or solutions
- improvised temporary works
- unfamiliarity with construction processes
- designs which create erection problems, eg connections
- inherent instability of structures prior to completion
- overloading incomplete or weak structures
- premature removal of temporary supports
- changing construction sequences
- uncoordinated site work/conflicting processes
- specification of hazardous materials

As a simple example, should the designer of a steel framed structure consider how components such as horizontal beams are to be connected within the flanges of vertical columns where the beam length is greater than the distance between the flanges? While there is no question that when complete the structure will accept all of the loads for which it is designed, failure to understand the practical problems of making the connections and to design a safe method could result in danger to erectors attempting to 'spring' or force beams into place while column fixings are slackened to allow movement and the structure becomes unstable. In fact, this scenario is typical of several real failures which have resulted in fatalities when structures have collapsed during construction, together with many other incidents where information on the inherent instability of partly complete structures could have been passed on by their designers. Solutions, such as the incorporation by design of shelf brackets and angle cleats, or of temporary bracings, are well known and readily available and good designers will make it their business to use them on the grounds that not only is safety improved but greater efficiency and cost-savings will be achieved.

As an example of a major incident, a collapse occurred in 1969 at the site of the Cleddau Bridge, Milford Haven, where an incomplete span of the massive steel-box girder failed while under construction. The report of the 'Inquiry into the Basis of Design and Method of Erection of Steel-Box Girder Bridges'(2) concluded unequivocally that the cause of the collapse was not inaccuracies in fabrication but that a steel plate diaphragm, an important element of the bridge box structure at the pier, was not strong enough as designed to resist the forces to which it was subjected while the span was being built incrementally outward as a cantilever. The important point that emerges is that while the bridge may have performed adequately as a completed structure, it had not been designed to take account of foreseeable erection loadings which, in the case of a bridge span to be built by that method, are very considerable and can induce stresses which are often greater and sometimes the reverse of those due to in-service conditions.

Closer to the main theme of this conference but still related to a design failure and with a construction element, in 1974 a massive explosion and extensive fires resulted in a heavy death toll, large numbers of injuries, wide-spread damage and huge financial losses at the Flixborough chemical works. The incident was found to have been caused by the failure of a connecting pipe bridging a gap where one defective reactor vessel had been removed from a line of six working at very high pressure and temperature as part of a refining process for cyclohexane, a highly explosive hydro-carbon product. Due to a difference in end levels of about 600mm, a cranked 500mm diameter steel pipe some 4m long was made up on site and connected at its ends to two 710mm diameter bellows attached to the adjacent reactor vessels. The pipe was supported by three cross-tubes of a light duty access scaffold and its end flange connections to flexible bellows on the reactors, but no design calculations had been carried out to determine loads on the scaffolding under full working pressure and temperature when the plant was put on stream again. The out-of-balance forces and massive rotational couple caused by the end reactions on the dog-leg pipe, which lacked restraint due to the flexibility of the end bellows and the purely nominal support of the scaffold tubes, resulted in failure of the bellows and release of a large aerosol cloud of material which detonated in the air above the plant, with disastrous effect. The lack of understanding of the forces which would be developed in the pipe and the failure to carry out a design and checking exercise for an engineered support, taking account of all of the loads developed, was the direct cause of one of the largest and most serious industrial accidents of recent years. It is significant that a major factor in the disaster was the decision to use light scaffolding erected by a local building firm without any formal design or information on eventual loadings or indeed of the load capacity of the framework.

THE INTEGRATED APPROACH - CDM AND ALL THAT

There is perhaps an element of arrogance in designers who consider construction problems to be the sole resonsibility of contractors and believe that they need have no involvement with or responsibility for the construction process, including safety, confining their interests to the delivery of completed structures. Fortunately, such attitudes are in the minority and most designers involved in construction work are competent and fully aware of the realities and complexities of site work. They take account of these factors in preparing their designs and provide suitable and adequate information for constructors, looking on this as a necessary feature of what is after all a partnership activity. By the same token, some clients and consultants procuring construction work distanced themselves entirely from any concern for safety, considering, as discussed above, that such matters were entirely the responsibility of contractors, based on the terms of their contracts and as required by criminal law.

Although, on the other hand, safety has been incorporated into projects as a necessary and integral component by many clients, consultants and designers for a very long time, concern grew over the accidents and losses in construction where this was not the case and eventually a European Directive gave rise to the Construction (Design and Management) Regulations 1994 (3), which formally imposed a statutory framework requiring the active participation of clients and designers in ensuring safety for construction work. The new Regulations could be said to have codified what more enlightened participants had been doing for a considerable time and we have only to look at the major power generation, petrochemical, chemical engineering and pharmaceutical industries to see examples of an enlightened and positive attitude to safety as an integral part of their projects. Perhaps a cynic might comment that with so much to lose if an incident occurs in one of their plants, then preventive measures make good commercial sense and a large investment in safety is a sensible move.

An excellent example of client-driven safety measures has been operating for some years, anticipating the CDM Regulations, at a major site being developed for a large multi-national pharmaceutical organisation. Clear and forceful requirements were laid down by the client for the site controls and safety procedures to be operated by their management contractor and sub-contractors, all of whose personnel had to undergo basic safety induction training before commencing site work. Among the measures introduced, in view of the high accident potential of site transport, was the introduction of a shuttle bus service between the individual construction sites on the project, coupled with a prohibition on any personnel walking on site access roads. Together with strict security measures to prevent unauthorised persons entering or moving about the very large site, accident levels have been minimal and hence losses are low and efficiency is high, an excellent example of the integrated safety approach and one method of creating a positive safety culture.

The application of the CDM Regulations to construction work created a certain amount of opposition in some quarters, particularly as the full realisation of duties imposed on clients and designers began to sink in. For the first time, clients were being required by criminal law to comply with wide-ranging demands to become deeply involved in construction work, amongst which was a responsibility to convey all relevant information about the condition of sites or premises where work was to be carried out. This was a major change from the days when tendering contractors would have to invest time and money in investigations which might not bear fruit if they failed to secure the contract and on reflection there is a great deal of good sense in the measure. Further, clients have the duty of ensuring the competence in health and safety matters of those they employ as Planning Supervisors – a new post required by the Regulations – as well as Principal Contractors and Designers, another sensible move.

It is the new duties and responsibilities of designers under the CDM regulations which constitute the most radical change from the former almost 'isolationist' position they occupied in relation to safety during construction. Whereas other parties involved in construction work are exempted from some provisions, designers seem to be liable for all their actions and it is they who are charged with 'avoiding foreseeable risks to the health and safety of any person carrying out construction or cleaning work or any other person affected'.

As regards their designs, they must ensure that they convey information about any and all residual risks to workers or others who may be affected, which of course includes the construction phase and would involve information about erection and instability problems, hazardous materials etc. If the CDM requirements on designers are properly implemented, it would appear that many of the items listed above as contributory factors to failures will be covered, either by their elimination as foreseeable risks, or, if this is not reasonably practicable – a process which must be capable of justification if required – then full information must be provided to limit risks.

The CDM Regulations are therefore seen as a blueprint for the creation of a legally imposed 'safety culture' where all the participants in construction work, from client through designers and main contractors to sub-contractors and the self-employed, are drawn into active and continuous involvement and responsibility for safety.

WAYS AND MEANS - MULTI-DISCIPLINARY SOLUTIONS FOR CONSTRUCTABILITY

With the application of the CDM Regulations to almost all construction work and the enhanced responsibilities of designers, as discussed above, methods are having to be developed by which designs are optimised for risk elimination and safe construction, in order to comply with the new requirements. A practical system which can be used to considerable effect is the establishment of a series of pre-tender 'constructability reviews'. These are meetings set up at appropriate intervals during the planning and design stages which are attended by representatives of all the professional disciplines and areas of activity involved in a particular sector of work at which the practical aspects of designs are discussed, including all the safety implications of the proposals. A typical early agenda would cover site clearance and demolition, excavations and foundations, calling for comments from section engineers, architects, and foundation specialists, also drawing on the expertise of environmental specialists if noise, dust and contaminated materials are involved. The benefit of such round table discussions is that problems are aired in front of all concerned and practical solutions can be reached more effectively than by individual meetings and paper studies in isolation.

Constructability reviews also provide a framework for CDM compliance by designers through assessment of their proposals in a pragmatic way by those who will be supervising construction. As an example, for construction of a bridge, the work site must be examined to ensure adequate space and load capacity to position cranes, access routes to bring in large articulated vehicles carrying precast bridge beams, locate existing services, examine ground conditions, storage for materials and other important site information necessary for inclusion in the health and safety plan to be provided with tender documents.

Additional meetings for a major project would cover structural engineering, cladding, roofing, mechanical and electrical services and fit-out, opening the way for any conflicts of interest or snags to be aired and solved at the earliest opportunity by discussion among those responsible for the various processes. By gathering expertise from a range of specialities in one meeting, a balanced view can be reached on the feasibility of all aspects of the proposed scheme or structure and safety considerations can be taken properly in context, which should ensure reduction of risks during site work by anticipating problems at an early enough stage and amending designs accordingly. When all that is reasonably practicable has been done to eliminate or reduce risks in designs, there will be the opportunity of ensuring that residual problems are the subject of adequate information in the health and safety plan, so that when tenders are returned, method statements for dealing with construction can be assessed.

A further advantage of such 'constructability reviews' is the creation of a team approach and, with careful management, a breaking-down of some of the inter-professional barriers which spring from differing interests and where construction work takes place under limited and difficult site conditions and constant pressure to expedite progress.

THE WAY FORWARD FOR DESIGN AND DESIGNERS

Within design organisations, there is a continuing need to provide effective training, supervision and encouragement of staff to inculcate a strong commitment to safety, where knowledge of the practical side of construction processes is part of their expertise. Unless designers are fully aware of the actual methods which will be used on site to assemble the components they have designed, including means of access and use of lifting equipment, problems will continue to be created for the work force and risks may exist which could have been eliminated on the drawing board.

The training of professionals must prepare them not only for the technicalities of their work, but also to be able to comply with legal requirements, at the same time serving the best interests of clients and constructors. To that extent, for the construction industry, the arrival of the CDM Regulations has formalised the need for an effective safety culture among designers by requiring deeper involvement and a wider knowledge of construction. While many practitioners have been operating on the lines of CDM for some time, the Regulations should now ensure that safety performance is improved across the board and no longer should those who give safety a high priority lose work to others who lack their commitment.

REFERENCES
1. Health and Safety Commission. Annual Report 1995/96. HSE Books, PO Box 1999, Sudbury, Suffolk CO10 6FS, 1996. ISBN 0 7176 1219 8
2. Department of the Environment. Inquiry into the basis of Design and Method of Erection of Steel-Box Girder Bridges. Report of the Committee, HMSO, London, 1973. ISBN 11 550279 3. 1973
3 Health and Safety Commission. Managing construction for health and safety. Construction (Design and Management) Regulations 1994 and Approved Code of Practice L54. HSE Books, PO Box 1999, Sudbury, Suffolk CO10 6FS, 1995. ISBN 0 7176 0792 5.

C537/005/97

The development of an operational safety culture

P McKIE CBE, DSc, CEng, FIEI, FRIC, FIQA, CIM, FInstD, CChem
DuPont, Bristol, UK

A complete operational safety system should encompass all aspects of technology, systems and culture. The author expands on the concept that, in industry, more attention is given to the technical and system aspects and too little attention is given to the people cultures necessary to ensure success. Some ways to redress this balance are discussed. The author draws heavily on his 38 years experience of operational management in E. I. DuPont de Nemours, a company with an enviable safety record.

1 ASPECTS OF SAFETY MANAGEMENT

A complete safety system will be part of an inclusive management system and will ensure that operations are technically sound, operated with systems that are complete and run by people who are knowledgeable and who apply that knowledge in a purposeful and consistent manner. This is illustrated in figure 1.

It is a fact, however, that management sometimes pays more attention to technology and systems than it pays to the people aspects of the operation. As is illustrated in figure 2 management frequently treats safety in a way which separates the technical aspects from the cultural aspects. This is unfortunate since, at least, in the experience of DuPont, the vast majority of injuries and incidents are caused by the unsafe acts of people. In DuPont 96% of all accidents and incidents are so caused (see figure 3). To achieve excellence in safety therefore attention must be given to developing a safety culture which recognises this fact and deals with it. This paper will therefore concentrate on the cultural aspects of safety. It is, of course, recognised that technology and systems are vitally important, however I plan to take this for granted and to discuss the people aspects almost exclusively.

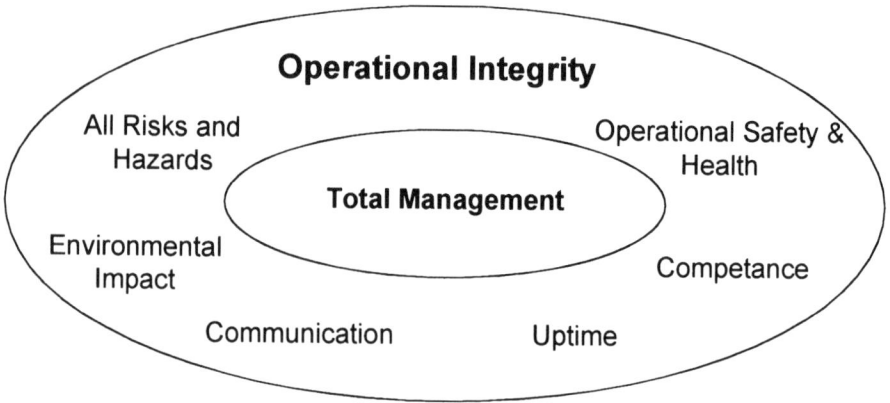

Figure 1. Inclusive Management System

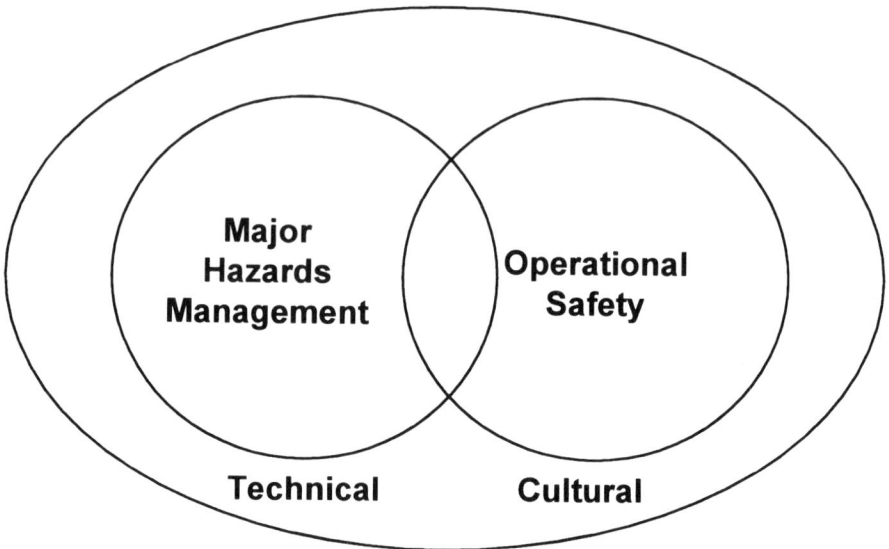

Figure 2. Total Safety Management System

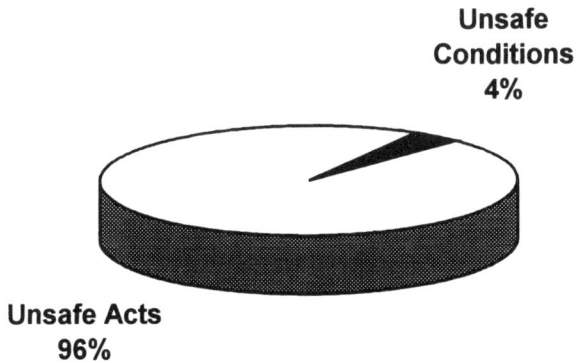

Unsafe Conditions 4%

Unsafe Acts 96%

Figure 3. Injury Causes

2 A SAFETY CULTURE

A definition of Culture from my dictionary is "The totality of socially transmitted behaviour patterns, arts, beliefs, institutions, and all other products of human work and thought". I believe this definition gives us the clues we need for the arrangements we need to make in an organisation to ensure success. In other words we need to have working systems that ensure people can interact one with the other in their work environment, and these interactions must allow for the people to have social intercourse and thoughtful discussions with their work groups, including the leadership teams.

All too often management believes that leadership in safety involves trying to provide a safe work place and endeavouring to police the actions of people to ensure they work safely.

This style of management will deliver a safety performance that is far from optimum for several reasons. For example:

A The possible positive contributions of many of the employees will not be sought or utilised.

B People may not work safely when management are absent.

C Management may well not have thought out all the possible problems that might be in the work place and may not therefore have an all encompassing process.

A much better management process will recognise the need for rules, regulations etc., but will provide a working environment, or culture, where each and every employee understands the need to work safely and ensures that they do so. They will also ensure fellow employees also work safely and will assist them in doing so without being asked to. We, in DuPont call this the "Brother's Keeper" concept. The challenge is how to cause this behaviour to become institutionalised in the organisation. In DuPont we have found that this culture is best developed in the following manner..

Firstly management must become determined to lead the whole process. It is a cliché to say it starts at the top, but frankly if it does not start there it does not start at all.

The steps that Management should take to achieve a high level of safety performance will be identical in concept to those it takes to manage all other aspects of the business. This is the first key point:
MANAGEMENT OF SAFETY IS CARRIED OUT JUST LIKE THE MANAGEMENT OF ALL OTHER ASPECTS OF THE BUSINESS.

3 MANAGEMENT OF SAFETY

A statement of the safety goal should be developed by the board. Since a goal is a long term expression of the aspirations of the company the goal should be challenging. At DuPont we believe that the only acceptable long term goal is for Zero injuries and incidents. This is founded on our belief that all incidents and injuries are avoidable, and that it is morally unacceptable to forecast that injuries will happen. As one strives to achieve that goal it will be necessary to establish improvement targets to track the progress towards the goal. Targets are, therefore, short term measurements of progress. A 50% year on year improvement target might be appropriate.

Management will also need to establish a safety policy for the organisation. Such a policy will be a clear statement of the values beliefs and expectations that management has for the organisation.

An organisation must be established to administer safety effectively, one that cascades from the top to the lowest levels in the business. This organisation must involve everyone and opportunities must be provided for groups to meet regularly to review progress against targets and goals, and to ensure everyone in the business has an opportunity to participate in the process.

Management must establish that the line organisation manages safety with safety professionals advising and guiding the process.

Management must set high standards of operational performance and insist that these standards are consistently met.

All of the above management processes, when established, will ensure that the climate in the organisation is one where safety is given it's appropriate priority . These processes might be thought of as establishing the rules for safe operation. They will show management's determination to achieve good performance. Such management determination will result in an improvement in the safety performance but it will not, on it's own deliver excellence in safety. A safety climate is not a safety culture.

The next step in developing the safety CULTURE must involve the wider workplace. The second key point to be made, therefore, is:
DEVELOPMENT OF A PROPER SAFETY CULTURE MUST INVOLVE THE PEOPLE IN THE WORKPLACE.

4 PEOPLE INVOLVEMENT

Bearing in mind the earlier statement that more than 90% of injuries in the workplace are caused by the unsafe acts of people, it is obviously vitally important to ensure that people work safely at all times. Whilst management can set rules and expectations for safe behaviour, supervision is not always present in the work place and therefore the behaviour of people must be managed by the people themselves. The challenge is how can we ensure that people behave in a safe manner at all times.

There is a popular misconception that people are risk averse. Nothing could be further from the truth. People are natural risk takers. We all take risks in our everyday life and we admire the risk takers in business and sport. The challenge, as we develop our safety culture, is to manage risk taking in a way that avoids injuries and incidents. People must accept their own responsibility for their safety in the work place and behave accordingly. Management can facilitate this acceptance in a number of ways. It might be appropriate to remind ourselves of the definition of culture. "The totality of socially transmitted behavior patterns, arts, beliefs, institutions, and all other products of human work and thought". People involvement is key to developing this culture. Some of the essential elements needed to develop this culture of people involvement flow from the definition.

Socially transmitted behaviour requires a high degree of communication. Such communication may be written or verbal but it must be two way communication. Of course management must direct communications and set directions, but management must also seek and react to, feed back. Frequently the shop floor personnel have ideas and opinions on safety that are additive to the process. Also, frustration will occur within the work force if they feel they are being ignored. This two way communication requires time and resources to be set aside to facilitate the process.

The transmission of beliefs requires a determined effort on the part of the whole team to ensure that commonly held principles and beliefs are well established. Again two way communication is essential in this process but this must be reinforced by training in interpersonal skills. Such training needs to be carried out throughout the organisation to ensure a common understanding and acceptance of the beliefs and principles of the whole team.

The last part of the definition refers to human work and thought. This implies that in all aspects of the work situation we must consider safety as part of the total environment. All decisions regarding the work situation must involve suitable regard for safety and safety must carry an appropriate priority. The safety culture will be irreparably destroyed if people are encouraged, or worse, directed to lower the priority given to safety when production, cost, or quality appear paramount. Safety must carry equal priority to these other parameters and people must behave in a manner that supports this equal priority.

The fact is, however, work is usually carried out by groups of people not individuals. Having people understand their individual responsibilities will not yet be enough to develop a truly successful culture. The third and last key point is therefore:
TEAMWORKING IS AN ESSENTIAL ASPECT OF A SUCCESSFUL SAFETY CULTURE.

5 TEAMWORK

Very few operations are carried out in the workplace by individuals. The vast majority of activity is done in a team environment, frequently in the absence of a formal leadership process. It is necessary, therefore, for management to ensure adequate training is given in the area of behaviour aspects of groups of people. People must be trained and encouraged to accept informal responsibility for tasks as they arise. Systems can be set up which give each team member a special area of responsibility and they can be trained accordingly. The team will then respond to the person with the special capability in a specific situation without regard for their hierarchical position. People must also accept that the priorities of the team transcend their own priorities and must be trained to behave accordingly. They will then accept responsibility for all their peers on the team. In this manner everyone is looking after their colleagues in a manner much more inclusive than by relying on direct supervision alone. This total process, when established, is what can be thought as a total safety culture.

6 SUMMARY

This total process is summarised on figure 4 which illustrates the cultural development of safety within an organisation in three phases.

If minimal regard is given for the safety process then people's natural instincts for self preservation will prevail. As previously stated this will result in an unacceptably high level of injuries. As supervision react to this in a mode of edict and control, by bringing in rules, ensuring adequate design for safety and carrying out basic training then the performance will improve.

As personnel develop their own beliefs around the need to work safely, and accept the safety culture and comply with the process to the best of their ability, then a further improvement in the performance will result.

The final step to developing a suitable safety culture, leading to the elimination of off injuries and incidents follows the establishment of a culture whereby everyone accepts the responsibility for themselves and everyone else in the organisation. In this mode, everyone will be constantly on the alert to ensure the behaviour of the whole team is constantly consistent with that required for a zero incident and injury performance.

Covey has described this development of individual responsibility a progressing from Dependence through Independence to Interdependence.

It is this interdependence state that is required for the ultimate safety process.

7 BENEFITS OF A TOTAL SAFETY PROCESS

It should be noted that in addition to the obvious safety benefits to an organisation which has achieved this interdependent behaviour significant other benefits accrue.

The need to do things in an orderly manner will positively affect cost, quality and customer service. In fact it will result in a considerable improvement of all business parameters.

8 EXAMPLES OF THE DEVELOPMENT OF A TOTAL SAFETY CULTURE

As examples that this approach does really work in the business world, figure 5 shows the safety performance of two plants bought as going concerns by DuPont in the late eighties. Both plants had been in operation for many years before acquisition, with safety performances typical of, or better than, UK equivalent operations.

Plant A is a Textile Fibre plant in the South of England and plant B has an engineering background in the North.

At both plants no significant changes were made to the technology and no new ideas were introduced regarding safety rules. Rather, emphasis was placed on developing, firstly, an independent culture with the employees and then a gradual transition was made to an interdependent culture. The results indicate that the process does in fact work. The business performance parameters also improved to the point that both sites attracted significant new investment and morale improved at both sites.

In conclusion I would assert that a safety performance of no injuries or incidents is achievable in industry, and that by following the processes described a CULTURE of safety management can be established which will deliver that performance.

9 COPYRIGHT

Copyright of this paper remains with the author P. H. McKie and DuPont UK Ltd.

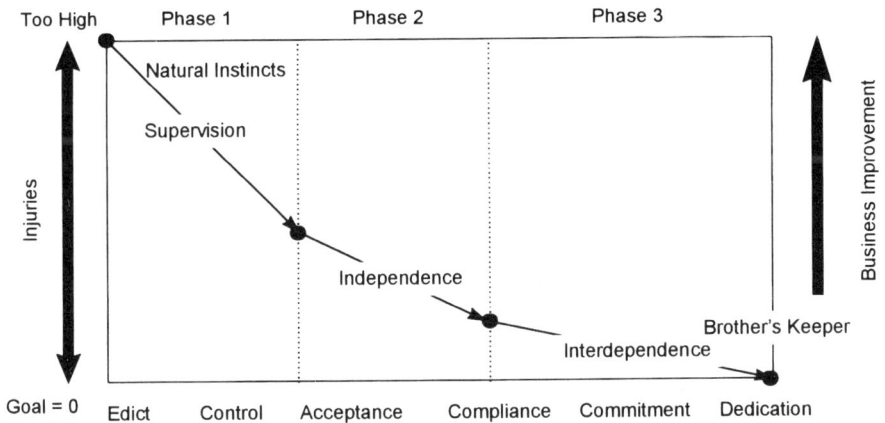

Figure 4. An Integrated Improvement Model

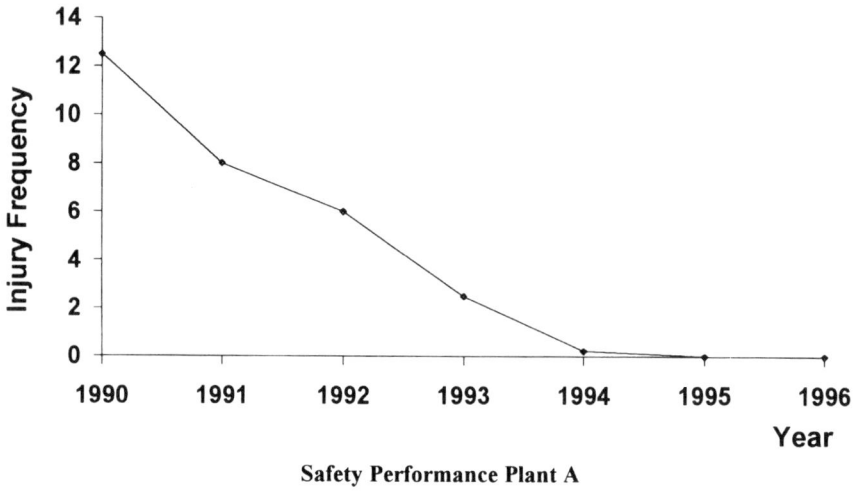

Safety Performance Plant A

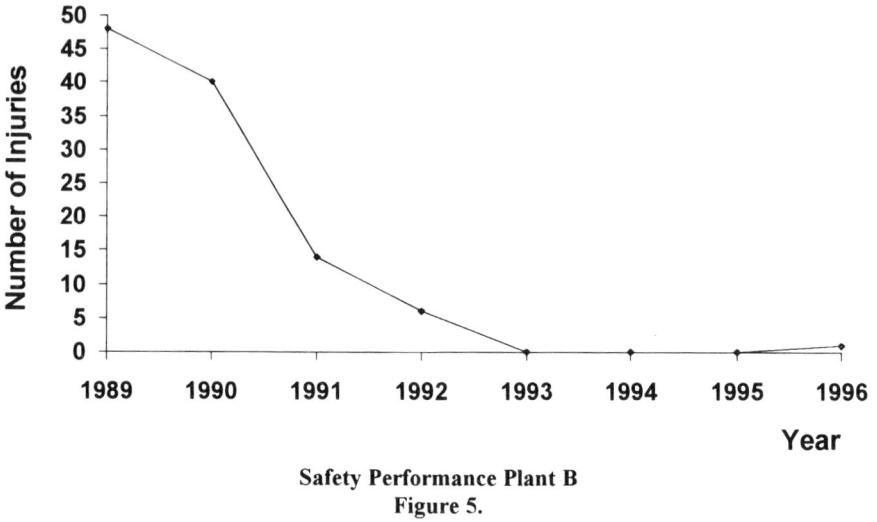

Safety Performance Plant B
Figure 5.

C537/006/97

Safety by design: an engineer's responsibility for safety

N JONES MSc, PhD, DSc, CEng, FRINA, FIMechE
Impact Research Centre, Department of Engineering, The University of Liverpool, UK

Synopsis
This paper provides some background material and motivation for a set of lecture notes which were produced recently by the Hazards Forum. This short course was developed specifically to provide an awareness of an engineer's responsibility for safety which could be incorporated into all undergraduate engineering programmes, regardless of discipline.

1. INTRODUCTION

The title of this paper is chosen deliberately as the title of a report published recently by the Hazards Forum (1). This paper discusses the background and objectives of this report and introduces the contents.

The Hazards Forum was set up in 1989 by the major engineering institutions as a result of a spate of major offshore, shipping, rail, air and flooding disasters within the U.K. It was soon realised that the Hazards Forum needed to focus part of its activities on the education of all chartered engineers to make them more aware of their responsibility for safety. Reference (2) was produced as a result of this concern and proposed a syllabus for a short awareness course which was designed to be suitable for all engineering disciplines. This document was circulated widely and views were obtained from a broad section of the engineering community, including the major engineering institutions. Subsequently, financial support received from National Power, The MacRobert Trusts and the Health and Safety Executive for the preparation of Reference (1). Reference (1) contains six major chapters forming the basis for lectures which aim to make all engineering undergraduates more aware of safety related matters.

Safety is, of course, a very complex area which is bound up with many issues such as economics, public perception, legislation and much else. Car safety, perhaps, illustrates some aspects of this complexity. It is estimated that about one-quarter of a million persons are killed worldwide each year in car accidents, as noted in the preface of Reference (3), and around ten times that number are injured seriously. Clearly, this carnage is acceptable to the general public, for, if it were not, then they would be willing to change their spending priorities to purchase safer cars, which can be built (4, 5), pay higher taxes to make roads safer, drive fewer miles, drive more slowly, or not at all.

Generally speaking, market forces are driving many systems to become larger (aircraft, lorries, buildings, bridges, etc.) and operate at higher speeds (transportation systems, engine components, etc.). Moreover, all engineering systems are being designed to use materials more efficiently with smaller associated margins of safety. All of these factors drive a design closer to a potential disaster in the event of a seemingly insignificant failure, unless proper cognizance is made of the various failure modes and adequate safety systems are incorporated during the design phase. Thus, it is as important as ever it was to consider safety matters in engineering notwithstanding the apparent sophistication of modern computerised design systems.

In addition to these observations, the general public is now much more aware of certain aspects of safety in the siting of industrial plant, transportation of hazardous materials, etc. Furthermore, legislation, including European, is becoming more onerous which acts as a brake on market forces by preventing cynical industrialists from operating systems that pollute the environment or cause an unacceptable number of injuries or even death in the unbridled pursuit of profit.

As the author writes this paper, some of these points are illustrated in a report which appeared in the Times today (6). An award of £2.1 x 10^9 was made to 8,000 people in New Orleans as a result of *"physical and mental injuries"* suffered when a rail tanker transporting a carcinogenic substance exploded in a marshalling yard near to an all-black residential area in 1987, the location of which led to the phrase *"environmental racism"*.

The foregoing remarks are made simply to acknowledge the complexity of this field. However, References (1) and (2) identify six major topics which all engineering undergraduates should have some awareness: Framework for Safety, Risk Modelling and Quantification, Legal Aspects of Health and Safety at Work, Cost and Acceptability of Risk, Human Factors in Health and Safety and Corporate Responsibility and Effective Management. It might well be asked, *"How can these subjects be taught within an already overcrowded undergraduate engineering syllabus"?* This is, of course, an important question, particularly in view of the poorer preparation in mathematics of many students entering universities in recent years which, inevitably, reduces the amount of material that can be covered in a typical engineering course. There are two possible replies, at least, to this question. One is that engineering courses should be at least four years long in line with Europe and the U.S. and preferably five years long, which is the duration of some non-engineering courses taught already in U.K. universities. The other response is that this field commands a high priority and that it is too important to omit. Its omission would be unfair both to a potential chartered engineer and to his/her potential employer as both might find themselves defending their actions in a court of law.

The proposed course of lectures, which are discussed briefly in the next section, require a minimum class room time of six hours and could be given at any time during an undergraduate engineering course. They could,with some advantage, be integrated into existing laboratory exercises, design courses, project work, etc.

2.   BRIEF SUMMARY OF THE SIX LECTURES IN REFERENCE (1)

2.1   Introduction

This section contains a brief introduction to each of the six lectures in Reference (1) which are designed specifically for an engineering undergraduate awareness course on responsibility for safety.

2.2   Framework for Safety

Professor R. Booth remarks that chartered engineers of all professional disciplines have an important role in ensuring the safety and health in many aspects of society. Their actions, or failure to act, can have a profound effect on people at work, within the home, on the road, in the air and in all systems involving technology and people. However, the concept of absolute safety is a myth since no system is totally safe.

Broad agreement exists within the community that the principles of safety management apply to the control of all hazardous events, no matter how diverse. Accidents generally do not have a single cause, but arise from the influence of many separate causal factors. Active failures are made by the people exposed directly to risk, while latent failures are those due to errors made by managers, supervisors, engineering designers and others in the organisational and technical foundations for hazardous events. In fact, it has been stated that each cause of a failure has two elements: a technical one, which leads directly to the failure, and a procedural one, which allows the faults to occur and go undetected and uncorrected.

Professor Booth discusses various matters including accident causation and prevention, proactive safety management and aspects of risk assessment. He concludes that accident prevention requires a combination of effective safety systems and professional competence. Successful systems rely on contributions from those directly at risk, as well as from managers and engineering designers.

This lecture forms a broad introduction to the remaining five chapters in Reference (1).

2.3   Risk Modelling and Quantification

Professor M. J. Baker has taken the subject of risk assessment introduced in Section 2.2 and developed it much deeper for use as a practical engineering tool. Particular attention is paid to concepts and terminology, the treatment of uncertainties and avoiding the temptation to regard risk and reliability as a property of the component or system alone. The probability of failure is not solely a property of the objective being assessed, but is a function of our state of knowledge of the object and the environment.

Professor Baker discusses risk modelling and quantification, which includes hazard identification and control, failure mode identification, methods for determining component failure probabilities and methods for determining system failure probabilities. Further comments are offered on modelling the consequences of engineering failures and risk quantification and control. In conclusion, it is remarked that the methods and controls introduced in this section must be used sensitively. A small engineering firm of a routine nature with relatively minor hazards requires a quantitative assessment of the physical hazards, but only a qualitative assessment, or ranking, of the associated risks. Projects with considerable potential for harming the workforce and/or general public require a fully quantitative risk assessment with the risks reduced to a level which is as low as reasonably practicable (ALARP, see Figure 1).

2.4 Legal Aspects of Health and Safety at Work

The third set of lecture notes in Reference (1), by Dr. D. Wenham, focus on the legal aspects of health and safety at work and identify the responsibilities under the current legal framework. Some attention is given to the influence of Europe on recent regulations.

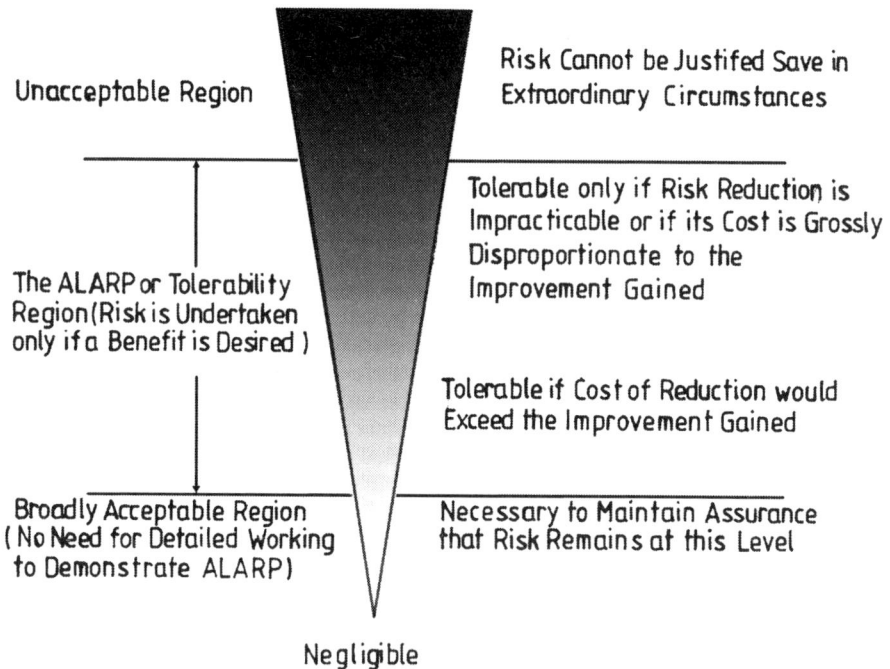

Unacceptable Region

Risk Cannot be Justifed Save in Extraordinary Circumstances

The ALARP or Tolerability Region (Risk is Undertaken only if a Benefit is Desired)

Tolerable only if Risk Reduction is Impracticable or if its Cost is Grossly Disproportionate to the Improvement Gained

Tolerable if Cost of Reduction would Exceed the Improvement Gained

Broadly Acceptable Region (No Need for Detailed Working to Demonstrate ALARP)

Necessary to Maintain Assurance that Risk Remains at this Level

Negligible

**Figure 1. Levels of Risk and ALARP
(as low as reasonably practicable) (1)**

It is remarked by Dr. Wenham that the legal basis for safety and health in the workplace is evolving rapidly as a result of pressures from within the U.K. and the European Union. In addition, people harmed in the work place are becoming more conscious of their rights and are seeking compensation in the courts, as noted already in §1. Chartered engineers of all disciplines play a major role in the conception, design and management of work place activities. Thus, they should be aware of the high legal standards expected from them and the consequences of failure to achieve them which results in an incident.

2.5 Cost and Acceptability of Risk

It is noted in §1 that the degree of safety that can be achieved in a given situation is bound up with cost. The design and manufacture of an extremely safe product might not be viable because it would be too expensive to capture a sufficient market share to cover costs and return a reasonable profit. This aspect of safety is addressed by Professor J. W. Reid in lecture 4 in Reference(1). He examines the economic and financial aspects of managing risk and safety and the trade-offs that need to be made between risk, which is discussed in §2.3, and cost.

An important point that must be addressed at the outset of this lecture is the acceptability of risk, which is a multi-faceted and complex topic, again as noted in §1. Generally speaking, safety law requires that any risk must be reduced to a level which is *"as low as reasonably practicable"*, or the ALARP principle illustrated in Figure 1.

The evaluation of risk in §2.3 is examined further by Professor Reid who considers such aspects as the cost of human life, the commercial impact of risk, the cost of risk control, cost benefit analysis and the financial control of risk.

2.6 Human Factors in Health and Safety

Professor S. Cox stresses the importance of human factors in health and safety in lecture 5 in Reference (1) because of the significant contributory role they play in safety issues. It is suggested that human factors are the underlying cause for up to 90 per cent of the accidents in recent years, possibly due, partly, to the enhanced reliability of technology.

Professor Cost introduces the topic of ergonomics and discusses various aspects including the Yerkes-Dodson law or the performance versus level of arousal curve in Figure 2. The form of this general relationship suggests that tasks should be designed to optimise individual performance. Anthropometry and biomechanics, physiology, psychology and human reliability engineering are other important topics which a chartered engineer should have some awareness in order to design safe systems and avoid unnecessary human stress levels and damage to health.

Two case studies illustrate the importance of human factors in the Three Mile Island nuclear power plant failure and in the space shuttle 'Challenger' disaster. Although these two disasters had many causative factors, human errors were involved at several levels in both cases, albeit of a different nature.

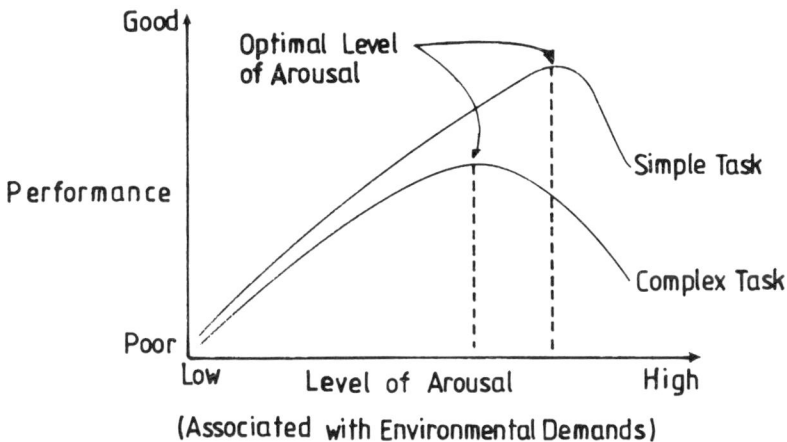

Figure 2. Performance versus Arousal Curve (1)

2.7 Corporate Responsibility and Effective Management

In the last lecture in Reference (1), Professor S. Dawson discusses the advantages and importance of integrating safety and health issues into corporate life, as illustrated schematically in Figure 3. Various criteria for assessing and improving effective health and safety management are introduced and illustrated including aspects of knowledge, motivation and organisational capacity. The safeguards required by an organisation which uses outside contractors is examined; an activity which has grown in recent years, and is known to have produced difficulties in some cases.

Professor Dawson devotes a final section to the actions which are required by corporations to achieve successful and effective health and safety management. It is stressed

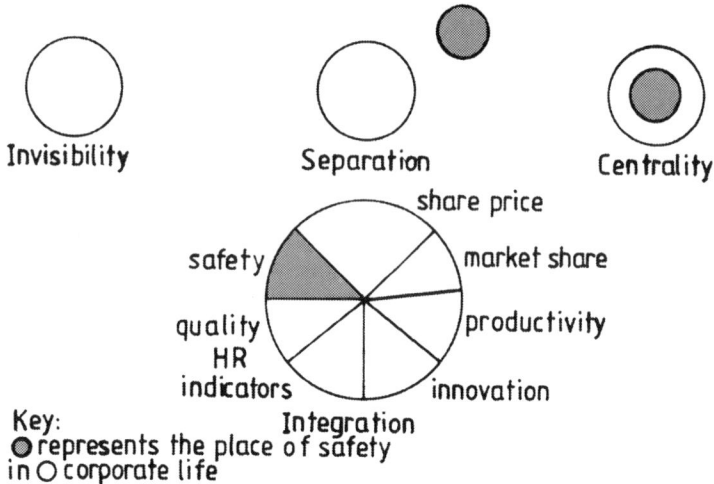

Figure 3. The Place of Safety in Corporate Life (1)

that the achievement of good performance in this area will not occur naturally, but only as the result of careful and considered investment in clearly identified goals and that all engineers have an important role to play in this matter throughout their professional careers.

3.   DISCUSSION

The six sets of lecture notes in Reference (1), which are discussed briefly in §2, were written by experts. Thus, they are authoritative and up-to-date introductions to the respective areas. However, it should be stressed that they are only introductions which are designed to provide all engineering undergraduates with an awareness of safety by design and its manifest aspects. Nevertheless, they are a gateway to deeper studies since all lectures contain a well chosen reference list.

It is important to note that accidents and disasters often have many causes, as brought out in the practical examples discussed by the authors, and as emphasised in the first set of lecture notes by Professor Booth (see §2.2). Thus, the topics in §2 and in Reference (1) must be integrated in practice and not considered in isolation.

It is likely that this whole area will continue to grow in importance because of the general trends noted in §1 and the consequent greater legislative activity and attendant regulation, partly from the European Union, and the increased tendency for injured parties to pursue litigation through the courts. Thus, it is vital to provide chartered engineers with some background and awareness in this general area. It is also important for chartered engineers to keep up-to-date with new developments throughout their career by attending courses and reading the appropriate literature produced by the Hazards Forum and other bodies.

It is proposed that this short awareness course, or an equivalent course, will become the minimum requirement for the accreditation of all undergraduate engineering courses in the U.K. and in Europe in the longer term. It is also necessary to produce an appropriate awareness course on safety for all technicians.

4. CONCLUSIONS

This paper provides some background and motivation for the set of lecture notes produced in Reference (1) for an undergraduate awareness course on an engineer's responsibility for safety. The six lectures are entitled framework for safety, risk modelling and quantification, legal aspects of health and safety at work, cost and acceptability of risk, human factors in health and safety and corporate responsibility and effective management. This introductory material is the minimum exposure to this important field which should become a requirement for all accredited undergraduate engineering degree courses, regardless of discipline.

These lecture notes are also suitable for engineers who did not have an opportunity to learn about these topics during their education and training.

ACKNOWLEDGMENTS

The author wishes to thank the many people within and outside the Hazards Forum, who have provided valuable ideas and assistance throughout the period from the initial meetings to produce the booklet cited as Reference (2) to the final set of lecture notes (1). In particular, he acknowledges Professors R. Booth, M. J. Baker, J. W. Reid, S. Cox and S. Dawson and Dr. D. Wenham who wrote the six chapters in Reference (1) which form the basis for my comments in §2.2 and §2.7 of this paper. The financial support of the Hazards Forum, National Power, The MacRobert Trusts and the Health and Safety Executive were vital to the success of this project and are gratefully acknowledged. Finally, I wish to record my appreciation to Mrs. M. White for her secretarial assistance and to Mr. H. Parker for his assistance with the figures, both from the Department of Engineering, Division of Mechanical Engineering at The University of Liverpool.

REFERENCES

(1)   "Safety by Design: An Engineer's Responsibility for Safety", 149 pp, ISBN 0
        952510316,1996.   Available from The Hazards Forum, 1 Great George Street,
        London, SW1P 3AA, price: £15.

(2)   "An Engineer's Responsibility for Safety: Proposed Syllabus for an Undergraduate
        Awareness Course", Hazards Forum, 7 pp, 1992.

(3)   Jones, N. and Wierzbicki, T., "Structural Crashworthiness", Butterworths, London,
        443 pp, ISBN O 408 01308 7, 1983.

(4)   Johnson, W. and Mamalis, A. G., "Crashworthiness of Vehicles", Mechanical
        Engineering Publications Ltd., London, 129 pp, ISBN 085298 386 7, 1978.

(5)   Murray, N. W., "When it Comes to the Crunch: The Mechanics of Car Collisions",
        World Scientific, Singapore, 164 pp,, ISBN 981 02 2096 0, 1994.

(6)   The Times, London, September 10, 1997.

C537/007/97

The application of fire hazard analysis

M GRANT BSc, PhD, MIMechE
W S Atkins Consultants Limited, Glasgow, UK

SYNOPSIS

The practical application of fire hazard analysis across the broad spectrum of industries is reviewed. Since Piper Alpha, the offshore oil and gas industry has applied fire hazard analysis on an unprecedented scale. This experience is drawn upon whilst recognising that the approach taken in other industries need not be as detailed given less complex and less hazardous operations.

The reasons for conducting fire hazard analysis in the first place are discussed. This is followed by a review of the steps that have to be taken to ensure that a competent analysis is produced. Finally the means by which a competent analysis can be translated into an effective action plan is considered. This last step ensures that the principal of reducing risks to a level that is as low as is reasonably practicable is achieved.

1 INTRODUCTION

The tools available to analyse the likelihood and consequences of fire are numerous and are increasingly more accessible. Importantly such tools are no longer necessarily the exclusive preserve of the expert in fire engineering. In theory therefore this should lead to wider and more beneficial use of fire hazard analysis. In practice this does not always occur for a variety of reasons. This paper is concerned with the steps that should be taken to ensure that fire hazard analysis is properly applied in practice.

In the aftermath of Piper Alpha we have seen the oil and gas industry radically change its perspective on the formal analysis of hazards. This has led, inter alia, to an industry wide application of fire hazard analysis which is unprecedented both in scale and in the associated acceleration in development of analysis technology. It is by no means suggested that a similar approach should be adopted in other industries. The offshore oil and gas industry is at the higher end of the risk spectrum and presents particular challenges from a technological viewpoint. Its techniques and methods for fire hazard analysis will therefore often be overly complex in the general industrial context. It is however entirely fair to suppose that some more general yet highly useful lessons can be drawn from the experiences of the oil and gas industry. It is from such a perspective that this paper is written.

It is important to bear in mind the regulatory background to fire hazard analysis. Various industries will have specific requirements in this respect but all undertakings must comply with the general principles embodied in the Management of Health and Safety at Work Regulations (1). Regulation 3 is quoted in part as follows:

(1) Every employer shall make a suitable and sufficient assessment of-

(a) the risks to the health and safety of his employees to which they are exposed whilst they are at work; and

(b) the risks to the health and safety of persons not in his employment arising out of or in connection with the conduct by him of his undertaking

This paper initially considers the benefits that can accrue from conduct of fire hazard analysis. The paper then goes on to consider two sets of issue in respect of the application of fire hazard analysis. One set is associated with ensuring that a competent fire hazard analysis is conducted in the first place. The other is associated with ensuring that the analysis is used in such a way that it positively improves the management of hazards in practice.

2 THE BENEFITS OF FIRE HAZARD ANALYSIS

It is as well to be completely clear about why fire hazard analysis is conducted. Fundamentally, it is to be recognised that unless the analysis ultimately affords the opportunity to change some facet of an operation then it is not worth doing. Sometimes fire hazard analysis is conducted as an end in itself and with the sole aim of demonstrating to some third party that a hazard management process is in place. In reality embarking on the analysis must imply a commitment to embrace its findings.

On a more positive note there are very many examples of how competent fire hazard analysis can improve not only safety but economic performance as well.

This is particularly the case during the design of an installation when fire hazard analysis has major potential for yielding benefit. Ideally conducted as early as possible the analysis should initially be used to improve the level of inherent safety. That is to say that at the earliest stages of the design the fire hazard analysis can identify areas where changes to the concept can give fundamental improvements in risk level. Examples of these are as follows:

- removal/minimisation of flammable materials
- keep flammables away from sources of ignition
- removal or reduction of sources of ignition
- segregate flammables from each other

- segregate flammables from locations where personnel are located
- for process plant, minimise the potential for release of flammables from their containment envelope

As the design develops, fire hazard analysis can be used to drive the design of fire protection systems such as detection, deluge, passive fire protection etc.. It can also influence issues such as development of operating procedures, maintenance strategy and emergency response planning.

Fire hazard analysis conducted on facilities that are already operating has a slightly different focus. The aim will be to augment an existing understanding of the hazards presented by the installation. This then can drive remedial work along the lines described above but is perhaps more likely to influence issues such as emergency response planning.

Above all else the fire hazard analysis will improve understanding of the risk picture. This allows appropriate risk management measures to be developed. In turn this permits lower levels of risk to be achieved. Furthermore the improved understanding of risk allows the use of the most appropriate technology. Fire protection systems thus need not be over specified hence economic performance can be improved. Similar arguments apply to the influence that fire hazard analysis has on operating procedures, maintenance strategy and emergency planning.

3 ACHIEVING COMPETENT FIRE HAZARD ANALYSIS

Personnel Competence

Self evidently, analysis conducted by incompetent personnel is not only useless but can be positively dangerous. This observation is however easily made and is not too helpful. More challenging is the issue of how competency can be assured. Were there a requirement for all fire hazard analysis to be conducted by specialists in the subject then competency would be relatively easily assessed. Qualifications, years of specialisation, peer group assessment might all be used to demonstrate that the specialist individual is competent. In short the same procedures as are applied for any other engineering discipline would be used.

Such an approach is right and proper but does not address the fact that if all fire hazard analysis were to be conducted by specialists then quite simply it would not all get done. The role of the specialist ought to be confined to those areas where a reasonable understanding of the hazards can only be achieved by application of in depth knowledge.

This then leads to the question of assessing the level of competence of the non-specialist. Many discipline engineers have a more than adequate competence in fire engineering which augments their core skills. This competence has however usually arisen through an interest in the subject including a substantial element of self-tuition. There is no shortage of high quality literature to support such endeavour. However only a few engineering degree courses contain any significant element of teaching on fire and related subjects. The availability of courses on fire hazard analysis, as opposed to the more general courses on risk assessment, is also limited.

There is thus a conflict which requires resolution. Of course, fire hazard analysis is better conducted by those who design or operate the installation. At present however it is rare for such persons to have even elementary training in the subject that would permit this goal to be realised. The provision of suitable training options would appear to be a priority.

Hazard Identification

If there is one factor above all others that determines the success of fire hazard analysis it would be the extent to which hazards are clearly identified. At one level hazard identification can be a fairly superficial exercise - the identified hazard associated with flammable material is generally fire. More meaningful is effort directed at identifying the causes and consequences of fire.

Understanding all of the potential causes of fire is necessary for proper management of the risks. Sources of ignition, accumulation of flammable material and other factors must be clearly and comprehensively identified.

Understanding all of the potential consequences is important to allow proper analysis of the fire to be conducted which in turn will allow proper identification of hardware and procedural measures for control of risk. The consequence picture will include consideration of some or all of the following:

- fire type (jet, pool, running, ventilation controlled etc.)
- thermal radiation levels
- smoke
- toxicity
- escalation to other flammable inventories, to structures or to adjacent areas
- collapse, missiles etc.
- threat to personnel in the vicinity, escape and evacuation routes and areas where people may muster

There are a number of means by which hazards can be identified. Checklists are often used to identify hazards but they raise question marks over the applicability of the list in particular applications and also the propensity of an individual to miss the obvious. The more successful identification techniques are those involving a group session with some element of brainstorming (2). This permits a much richer identification process capitalising on the way in which different perspectives can combine to reveal hitherto unrecognised sequences of events that can lead to a hazard.

Timing

The author's experience is that very few fire hazard analyses are later condemned as having been conducted too early. Those that fall into the category of having been conducted too late are far more numerous. During the design stage of an installation 'too late' will mean that the opportunity to influence the design in an economic manner has been lost. For an operating installation too late will mean that important knowledge regarding hazard management is not available and hence the operator may not be discharging due responsibilities under the MHSWR (1).

The analyses conducted at the earliest stages of the design process when only the sketchiest of detail is available are potentially the most useful as it as this stage when there is most leverage on the design process as has been discussed earlier.

As early as possible is thus the recommendation with respect to timing. The only proviso is that it is important to monitor the ongoing design to ensure that assumptions made previously remain valid and adherence to recommendations made previously remains in place. The rationale behind good thinking during the early stages of a project can easily become lost

C537/007 © IMechE 1997

in the mists of time. It should also be noted that as the project progresses, fire hazard analysis with a different focus becomes necessary. As an example a quick and early fire hazard analysis might have determined that application of passive fire protection was the preferred and most cost effective risk control strategy. Later analysis once the size of flammable inventories was fully known might be required to permit proper specification of the passive fire protection.

Review Cycle

Fire hazard analysis can not be seen as a one off exercise as all industrial operations are subject to change and this may introduce new hazards or modify those that already exist. It is important therefore that that fire hazard analysis is reviewed on a regular basis. It is suggested that this should be conducted on two bases:

- a regular review cycle, for example on an annual basis
- a review triggered by changes in the operation of the undertaking

In this manner the analysis can considered to be 'live' and hence a true representation of the risk picture.

Level of Detail

Deciding on an appropriate level of detail for the analysis has major influence on the success of the final outcome. Application of numerical combustion models can imply a significant cost and time penalty (although this is less the case than it once was). This will render their use inappropriate for very many industrial applications not least because relevant risk reduction measures under consideration may cost less than the analysis itself. On the other hand high risk installations may well imply high cost risk reduction measures and the additional insight provided by more detailed analysis is likely to be cost beneficial. Examples of this latter category include offshore oil and gas installations, refineries, petrochemical plant, underground railways, nuclear power stations, some high occupancy buildings and so on.

The hazard identification exercise as discussed above will go a long way to allowing initial assessment of complexity and level of risk. This in turn will allow judgments to be made about the necessary and justifiable complexity of the fire hazard analysis.

4 TRANSLATING ANALYSIS INTO ALARP

Assessment

Assessment is the process by which the analysis is translated into an action plan. The fire hazard analysis will probably lead to some recommendations but these may be quite generalised and with the best will in the world are formed from what may be the limited perspective of the analyst. For the analysis to have proper leverage on the risk picture it is necessary to translate recommendations into specific actions. This must be done taking into account the wider operational and design constraints.

The assessment process should thus be conducted by a broad group of personnel which can include the following:

- discipline engineers
- operations staff
- fire risk specialists
- management

Give that this group are committed to the common view that risks should be reduced to a level that is as low as is reasonably practical the assessment process will lead to a set of focused recommendations. These may encompass design and procedural changes and in some instances may involve doing nothing if the status quo is judged satisfactory.

Implied in this process is that the assessment team have the authority to initiate actions. This might additionally require some higher level of review or approval but the key is to be clear about the executive processes from the outset.

Tracking

The assessment process is likely to lead to a series of recommendations. In order that these are carried through to implementation it is vital that some form of recommendation tracking system is put in place. The key facets of the system are as follows:

- assignment of ownership
- recording of timescales for action
- implementation of a review cycle
- close out

At the simplest level where only a limited number of recommendations are involved, the tracking process need not be too involved and can probably be incorporated into some existing framework such as a regular Site Safety Meeting. A more complex fire hazard analysis will tend to generate more recommendations and some form of formalised computer tracking system is probably justified.

Timing

The need to set timescales for any corrective action was raised above. It is important to note that reduction of risks to a level that is as low as is reasonably practicable also implies an imperative to implement corrective action as soon as is reasonably practical. Time for due consideration of all of the implications of any action is justified as is scheduling work such that it does not in itself pose a hazard. Excessive procrastination is however as much a breach of legislative and moral duty as taking no action at all.

5 CONCLUSIONS

The hazards arising from fire can only be properly controlled if they are well understood. A fire hazard analysis conducted at an appropriate level of detail for the facility in question is an essential step in the process.

The key success factors that ensure fire hazard analysis is conducted properly are the competence of the analyst, thorough hazard identification, doing the analysis at the right time and selecting an appropriate level of detail for the analysis. Of these competence is the most problematic issue. Fire engineering experts will meet competence criteria but may not always represent the most appropriate solution. Discipline engineers have the familiarity with the facility but rarely have adequate training in fire engineering. The situation could be improved by wider provision of training in fire engineering.

To translate the analysis into better risk management it is important that sufficient weight is given to assessing the findings of the analysis. This means involving a suitably senior and broad group of personnel in the process. It will also mean having a formal tracking process for any recommendations that arise which should in turn ensure that required change is implemented in a reasonably timely manner.

6 REFERENCES

(1)   Management of Health and Safety at Work Regulations 1992
(2)   Can We Identify Potential Major Hazards, Crawley, FK, Grant, MM and Green, MD, IChemE Symposium Series No 130, Manchester 1992

C537/008/97

Fire hazard analysis techniques

K CASSIDY MA, MSc, MInstChemE
Health and Safety Executive, Merseyside, UK

Summary

This paper, considers, very briefly,
* the role of regulation in risk management
* the locus of QRA in risk management
* relevant hazard and risk assessment methodologies
* uncertainties in the risk assessment process
* modelling complexities
* some current needs in fire and explosion modelling

1. INTRODUCTION

The role of regulation, and that of the regulator, has recently been addressed by Rimington (1); and in that analysis he addresses some of the tools available to the regulator, including the use of risk assessment as a component of risk management. Not surprisingly, there is no agreed definition of 'risk management' - the issues involved may be very complex - but it is possible to characterise the overall process into a coherent overall architecture, based on the principles of

-	IDENTIFICATION	-	the recognition and location of any potential problem;
-	ASSESSMENT	-	the bounding and dimensioning of any potential problem;
-	CONTROL	-	the limiting of the scale of any potential problem, by prevention or avoidance;
-	MITIGATION	-	the amelioration of the residual elements of the potential problem.

This is a strategy first applied, in the UK, to the control of major chemical hazards as a result of the recommendations of the UK Advisory Committee on Major Hazards (2) but it is an overall approach which is universally applicable. Measures used to parameterize, or to limit, the component elements may vary between hazards and risks, between different components of the overall environment, or between different economic and cultural systems;

but the underpinning logic of the approach remains as a taxonomy comprising overall environment, or between different economic and cultural systems. (3)

2. GENERAL PRINCIPLES FOR RISK CRITERIA

The framework on which risk control is based in the UK is described in HSE's document on the tolerability of risk from nuclear power stations (2) - a publication which addresses issues far wider than its title would imply. The framework reflects well established approaches in international risk control, particularly related to advanced, high technology activities, such as those of the nuclear industry, the latter being expressed in the 1977 Report of the International Commission on Radiological Protection (3). The ICRP recommendations embodied the interrelated principles of justification of practice, optimisation of radiation protection, and individual dose limits. No practice or activity involving exposure to radiation was to be adopted unless its introduction produced a positive net benefit in a society, this benefit to be maximised by the 'as low as reasonable achievable (ALARA)' principle, and inequitable distribution at the level of the individual avoided by dose limits for that individual.

Such principles apply, of course, to the control of most risks. In an ideal world, any hazardous activity would not impose risks which were disproportionate to the benefits (such benefits come from a wide spectrum, and inevitably involve economic as well as other, often less tangible, social value parameters), and any such risks would be equitably distributed amongst society in proportion to the benefits received. In practice, of course, such distribution is not possible, and the principles of distribution described above are applied in a more general way, involving tests to ensure:-

a)   whether a given risk is so great, or the outcome so unacceptable that it must be refused altogether; or

b)   whether the risk is or has been made so small that no further precaution is necessary; or

c)   if a risk falls between these two states, that it has been reduced to the lowest level practicable, bearing in mind the benefits flowing from its acceptance, and taking into account the costs of any further reduction.

These principles combine with other generally accepted tenets:-

d)   that risks should never be imposed unnecessarily; and

e)   that no individual or community should bear an unfair proportion of any risk

to form the basis of UK Health and Safety law, that any risk must be reduced 'so far as is reasonably practicable' or to a level which is as low as is reasonably practicable - the ALARP principle. It is a principle which applies whether the need for risk control is expressed in qualitative terms (as, for instance, in regulations such as COSHH (4) or in the UK embodiment of the CEC Framework Directive (5) or by various quantified approaches, (usually involving QRA) applied in more complex 'risky' activities; and it contains an additional dimension (the test of 'gross disproportion' (6)) to those judgements involved in cost benefit, or cost effectiveness analyses.

The general structure of this mechanism of control is now well recognised and accepted; and it is an overall approach applicable equally to both 'individual' and 'societal' risks control.

(**NOTE:** individual risk: the frequency at which an individual may be expected to sustain a given level of harm from the realisation of specified hazards)

Societal risk: the relationship between frequency and the number of people
suffering from a specified level of harm in a given population from
the realisation of specified hazards.

These being the definitions in the 'nomenclature' document of the Institution of Chemical
Engineers (7). However, HSE has suggested other definitions (8).

It is, however, a conceptual framework. And it is for a regulatory or other control body to
propose criteria for what should be judged acceptable, tolerable, intolerable, negligible, trivial
etc; the outputs of QRA supply only one technical input into an arena of decision making in
which value judgements of one kind or another are central.

Such value judgements involve very complex social processes. Hazards and risks are
viewed quite differently, depending on the origins of the hazards and the nature of the risks
they present. Natural hazards seem to be 'accepted' more readily than those which are man
made; and hazards which presage catastrophe appear less 'acceptable' than those presenting a
lower level, continuous risk. A relatively well established hierarchy of 'tolerability' has
emerged, which involved issues such as:-

- voluntary vs involuntary exposure
- 'natural' vs man-made risks
- perceptions of personal control
- familiarity
- perceptions of benefit or disbenefit
- the nature of the hazard or consequence
- the nature of the threat
- the special vulnerability of 'sensitive' groups
- public perception of the extent and type of risk
- perceptions of comparators
- the reversibility of effects.

It is a decision hierarchy which turns on the confidence of those exposed to the risks in
those authorities and bodies who create and control the risks - government, the regulatory
authorities, plant operators, 'experts', and emergency services. Priority questions include:-

-          does the public believe that all views and interests have been considered in the
decision making process, or has there been some 'dealing'?

-          does the public have confidence in the effectiveness and independence of the
regulatory authorities?

-          is there a consistent and credible consensus of scientific opinion about the project that
the public can trust, or do the 'experts' disagree amongst themselves?

-          what is known about the quality of the project and plant management?

-          are the emergency and medical services able to cope with any event, in the short or
long term?

It is, in effect, a combination of physical and social detriments, in which some major
elements may not be quantifiable in any meaningful way.

3. THE ROLE OF RISK MEASUREMENT IN THE COMMUNICATION OF RISK

A major role of (Q)RA is the effective communication of the risks involved. Covello (9)
identified 19 characteristics of risk which must be considered in QRA applications if there is to
be sufficient information for evaluating these risks and making appropriate decisions. These
characteristics can be grouped under three major headings

- perspective on risk, which refers to ways in which risks are viewed by users and decision makers within the context of the problem being addressed
- criteria for measuring risk, which refers to analytical output from QRA
- relevance to decision making, which addresses the broader issue of the ability of QRA to advise on an appropriate course of action.

Most QRA models express individual risk as the probability of a stated detriment (often death) per unit interval of time, often in terms of equal probability isopleths, etc. Societal risks are, however, more complex, being normally expressed either as an expectation of harm (often death) or as a plot of the frequency of N or more deaths per unit time versus the number of deaths. This latter more complete representation of societal risk is the cumulative F-N curve. Societal risk expectation is simply the expected value of the F-N curve.

There appears to be some consensus that FN curves, despite their complexities, uncertainties, and difficulties, currently offer the best means of expressing societal risk. However, various commentators have suggested ways in what the curves can be better represented. These include

a) the use of probability density functions and probability of exceedance curves (Bernouilli, exponential, and inverse quadratic), which Vrijling et al (10) merge, into a simple theory of acceptability, two specific Dutch approaches

b) extending the range of consequences reflected in the F-N relationship, to include other consequence measures - especially as these may affect different mitigating responses. The measures could include personal injury, property damage, environmental impact, and relate to both short term and long term harm

c) using alternative ways of defining risk consequences. Here the probability of incurring fatality in the F-N curve requires an additional step in the analysis to translate 'exposure to dose' to 'fatality response', normally using a probit dose-response formulation, in which the input dose (expressed as a function of concentration and exposure time) becomes an input to a public expression, with the dependent variable being a measure of the probability of death

d) linking F-N curves to mitigation. This can include mitigation measures at both the individual level and at the level of official or other response

e) including monetary factors. In real terms, decisions are rarely made in the absence of financial considerations (ie. the cost of mitigation vs the benefits of risk reduction). This approach requires the risk output to be reported in such a way as to permit a thorough cost effective valuation of alternative forms of mitigation. It could involve assigning values to deaths, injuries and property values in the F-N curves and assessing the costs of alternative types of mitigation, including emergency response (inc. evacuation), containment, and clean-up, as well as risk avoidance. Some current research work by Keller & Cassidy (11) is providing useful insights into the potential of this approach, converting accident and other data to logarithmic magnitudes and analysing using Maximum Likelihood, with exponential Weibull, and a specialised Weibull, probability distribution analysis

f) expressing uncertainty in the F-N relationship. Because uncertainty in risk estimation varies with the number of reported cases used in validating the model estimates, the uncertainty associated (for example) with very low frequency/high consequence events is likely to be greater than the uncertainties in the reverse case. Accordingly, certain regions of the F-N curve are more prone to uncertainty than other regions, and this should be taken into account in representing the results. The normal procedure for this is to establish confidence limits about each point on the F-N curve. Of course, imperfect information will always produce risk estimates that are subject to error. True values of risk are unlikely ever to be known. Confidence bands in F-N curves are helpful to decision makers because they provide a range of values within which the true value of risk lies, with a percentage level of confidence. The bands can also serve as a basis for comparing uncertain estimates from different sources

g) use of expectation values. Frequently, societal risks in F-N curves are combined over all consequent damages and expressed as a single damage value (e.g.. expected fatalities per year). On occasion, such use of expected values has created problems for validation of QRA models and has fostered a belief that these models are unnecessarily alarmist when compared to historical experience. This leads to a need for caution in using and interpreting QRA results based exclusively on the expected value of harm, especially when historical data may have been collected over an inappropriate time period, or the work is subject to a significant latency period.

Other quantified approaches are currently being developed for addressing aspects of societal risk. These include

(i)   the use of expected (dis)utility criteria (12), which offer some advantages (but with concomitant disadvantages) over F-N curves

(ii)   a Risk Integral and Scaled Risk Integral approach (13). This approach is very useful in specific local cases, but is limited or not applicable in wider application.

4. RISK MANAGEMENT AND ALARP

Risk Management, put at its most simple, addresses the key questions
WHAT IF?
WHAT THEN?
THEN WHAT?
SO WHAT?

'What if?' requires a combination of technical expertise, experience, and a degree of imaginative insight. 'What then?' and Then What?' are essentially the techniques and practices of risk assessment. 'So What?' is the area of judgement, informed but not constrained by the earlier inputs. It is a decision process, often rigorous, which involves:-

a)   quantification of likely risk with an understanding of the inherent uncertainties involved in the assessment process

b)   reference to the likely benefits generated and the political and economic considerations associated with it

c)   judgements as to tolerability or acceptability for groups directly of indirectly affected; and

d)   sometimes, decisions as to further reductions in risk taking cost (including effort, and available technology) into account.

It is, in short, a process which is essentially economic and political, technically informed. It involves an interactive process addressing (using risk assessment jargon)
the SOURCE
the SOURCE TERM
the DISPERSION
the DOSE
the IMPACT
in which there are many common components, including
- in identification: the use of a substances/threshold approach (and the importance of search for a hazard or risk equivalence system);

- <u>in assessment</u>:   the classical approaches to consequence and probabilistic assessment. These include

(i)   Comparative methods, such as
   - Process/system checklists
   - Safety Audit/Review
   - Relative Ranking (e.g. Dow and Mond Indices)
   - Preliminary Hazard Analysis
(ii)   Fundamental Methods, such as
   - Hazard and Operability Studies
   - 'What if' Analysis
   - Failure Mode and Effect Analysis
   - Failure Mode, Effect, and Criticality Analysis
(iii) Logic Diagram Methods
   - Fault Tree Analysis
   - Event Tree Analysis
   - Cause Consequence Analysis
   - Human Reliability Analysis
   - System Success Trees

An essential element of the above, or similar methods, is provided by consequence assessment and analysis. Such processes involve modelling of the chemical and physical phenomenology associated with

- discharge types and rates
- aerosol effects
- evaporation
- dispersion (whether buoyant, passive, or dense)
- thermal radiation, including
   - flash fire or cloud fire
   - jet fire
   - pool fire
   - fireball/BLEVE
   - ventilation controlled fires
- explosion effects (over pressure, projectiles, etc)

(Dr Martin Grant will address in detail some of the models associated with such analysis, in a subsequent paper at the conference).

- <u>in control</u>:   the application and enforcement of technical, operational and legal standards;
            information and descriptive packages (e.g. the 'safety report' approach)
            descriptive and analytical system justifications (the 'safety case' approach);
            licensing approvals or other ways of granting permission
- <u>in mitigation</u>:   on site emergency planning;
            off site emergency planning;
            information to those who may be affected by the risks;
            controls over incompatible land use;
            siting controls for risk sources.

QRA, in all these areas, has the capacity to dimension, to rank, to focus, and to test the interdependence and interactive response of component elements.

There are, of course, many uncertainties
- in the identification process, where lack of comprehensiveness may induce critical error
- in the assessment process, where, despite continuing major research, uncertainties still remain in such areas as
  the selection of failure cases from the range of possibilities
  failure probabilities for each failure case
  scale of release rates and duration
  conversion of a failure case to a source term for use in further calculation
  the validity of the dispersion model
  meteorological inputs
  topographical inputs
  human and environmental response to toxic, pressure, or thermal burdens
  ameliorating factors
  ignition factors
  and in particular
  parameter values in many of the mathematical models.
- in the evaluation process, where the socio-political issues summarised in Section 2 above are paramount.

In many cases, sensitivity testing can be of immense value not only in assessing the effects of uncertainties, but in identifying critical areas of control; and adding insight to the tolerability debate and the validity and relevance of the criteria applied.

5. CURRENT NEEDS IN FIRE & EXPLOSION MODELLING

In the past 15-20 years, very considerable effort has been deployed in the development of relevant technical models in the areas of
- preventative technologies
- chemical and physical phenomenology
- risk mitigation and risk management

with the greatest effort probably in the phenomenology area. Indeed, it is arguable that in a number of such areas, the potential for further improvement in practical tools, (as opposed to the further clarification and development of the concomitant science), is of only limited cost benefit. And for this it follows that any further significant deployment of further resources in these areas must be carefully focussed.

In the opinion of the author, the areas below are the areas of remaining uncertainty which should receive priority attention, in any future work.

(a) Scaling Verification and validation of models by and against larger scale experimental (or well documented accidental) releases

(b) Source Terms Verification and validation of simplified models, including release state

(c) Dispersion dispersion in low and very low windspeed, wake effects, dispersion in complex arrays and terrains

(d) Fires
  (i)   Pool - Products of incomplete combustion
  (ii)   Jet - Non-sooting flames
  (iii) Compartments - Effects of lack of ventilation
  (iv)   Cloud - Flame front propagation
  (v)   on water - Surface mobility and spread

(e) <u>BLEVE</u> large scale effects
(f) <u>Explosions</u>
     (i)   combustion explosion, development in unconfined structures
     (ii)   vented. Effects of venting
     (iii)   explosion scaling
(g) <u>Computational fluid dynamics</u> Cost effective application and use
(h) <u>Direct Numerical Simulation</u> vs experimental data
(i) <u>Response of structures</u>
     (i)   to fire
     (ii)   to explosion
(j) <u>Human Response</u> elements of mitigation

6. MODELLING COMPLEXITY

Of course, there are many levels of complexity in consequence analysis, within the following range:-

a) simple threshold - e.g. consequences of most foreseeable event

b) qualitative analysis of releases - e.g. Risk of events, combined with level of protection: one or two dominating events

c) historical - e.g. based on analysis of similar installations, plus analyses

d) quantitative analysis of releases, frequencies - e.g. list of events, size, frequency leading to overall risk figure

e) quantitative synthesis - event trees -> significant events, fault trees - quantity, frequency, leading to overall risk figure

And of course, with increasing size and complexity, there is a concomitant increase in resource cost, and uncertainty.

7. SUMMARY

This paper has briefly addressed the locus of consequence and risk assessment approaches in the overall process of risk management and risk tolerability. It has considered the basic assessment tools and approaches currently available and identified areas of importance for further research and developmental work.

'REFERENCES'

1. Coping with Technological Risk: A 21st Century Problem. JD Rimington. Engineers & Society: the 1993 CSE Lecture.
2. Advisory Committee on Major Hazards; Three Reports 1976, 1979, 1984.
3. 'Risk Management: a business risk or a risky business?' K Cassidy. American Institute of Chemical Engineers/Center of Chemical Process Safety. San Francisco, September 1993. ISBN 0-8169-0589-4.
4. Control of Substances Hazardous to Health Regulations 1988. HMSO.
5. Directive 89/391/EEC. OJEC 1989.
6. Edwards v National Coal Board (1949) 1 AER 743.

7. Institution of Chemical Engineers: Nomenclature of Hazard and Risk Analysis in the Process Industries. I Chem E London. 2nd Edition 1992.

8. Generic Terms and Concepts in the Assessment and Regulation of Industrial Risks. HSE discussion document 1995.

9. Covello, V.T. Prospects and Problems in Risk Communication (Leiss, ed.) University of Waterloo Press, Waterloo, Ontario, Canada, 1989.

10. 'What is acceptable risk?' J.K. Vrijling. JFM Wessels, W van Hengel, R.J. Houben. Directoraat General Rijkswaterstaat. Report No BSW 93-23.

11. Analysis of fatality, evacuation, and cost data using Bradford Disaster Scale Magnitudes. Cassidy K and Keller A.Z. (AIChE/CCPS International Conference and Workshop on modelling and mitigating the consequences of accidental releases of hazardous materials. New Orleans. September 26-29 1995).

12. What is wrong with criterion F-N lines for judging the tolerability of risk? Evans A.W. and Verlander N.Q. Conference on Risk Analysis and Assessment Institute of Mathematics and its applications, University of Edinburgh, 14-15 April 1994.

13. The Scaled Risk Integral - a simple numerical representation of case societal risk for land use planning in the vicinity of major accident hazards. Carter D.A. (presented to the 8th International Symposium on Loss Prevention and Safety Promotion in the Process Industries), Antwerp, 19-23 June 1995.

C537/010/97

Fire and explosion hazard management in the chemical and hydrocarbon processing industry

F K CRAWLEY BSc, ARCST, FIChemE
W S Atkins, Glasgow, UK
G A DALZELL BSc, FIMechE
BP Exploration, Aberdeen, UK

<u>Synopsis</u>

The paper describes the way in which Fire and Explosion Hazards are managed in the Chemical and Hydrocarbon Industry. It outlines the evolution from the prescriptive legislative regime to a goal setting culture in which the assessment of hazards is used as the basis of design and operation. The life cycle approach to hazard management as developed for the offshore industry is recommended as a structured way of ensuring that all hazards are effectively and economically managed. Finally, it advocates that prevention, rather than protection should be encouraged as the primary means to reduce fire and explosion risks.

1. INTRODUCTION

The materials handled in the Chemical and Hydrocarbon processing industry are an ever present source for potentially catastrophic fires and explosions. Large oil refineries may handle over 100,000 tonnes of highly flammable fluids per day and, providing these are contained wholly within the equipment, nothing usually occurs. Some of the causes are special to the industry, such as runaway chemical reactions or detonation arising from the fluids and gases that are processed. In other ways, however, there are similarities with other industries. There are power stations, switchgear, warehousing, control rooms and, in the offshore industry, airports and hotels. Above all, there are people who make mistakes and people who get killed.

Some of those mistakes have included:

- Flixborough UK; 28 killed   (1)
- San Juan Ixhuatepec Mexico City; ca. 550 killed   (2)

- Los Alfraques Spain; ca. 200 killed   (3)
- Piper Alpha UK; 167 killed   (4).

There have been mistakes in the design and operation of particular plants, and in the whole approach to the management of fire and explosion hazards. It is not to say that the petrochemical and offshore industry was not trying to be safe, but it may not have been trying hard enough, and certainly its efforts may not have been focused on the right hazards or on the most effective ways of reducing them.

The industry has changed and should share both its mistakes and lessons learned, with other industries.

2.   THE HAZARDS

Within the industry, the release of a fluid may result in a fire or explosion. Most processing works in a steady state with flow rates, temperatures and pressures remaining constant. Materials enter the process, go through exactly the same operations, in the same physical conditions and then leave the process. Unlike other industries, a time lapse photograph taken in the plant or control room would show little change over 365 days a year. Occasionally there will be subtle changes for maintenance, modification, process upset conditions or start-up and shutdown.

It is also a highly controlled environment with site access limited to authorised personnel and work only carried out by competent people under the appropriate control. It should be easy to identify who is on site, where they are and what they are doing. With such a controlled environment, the range of credible major hazards is limited and they should be easily identifiable. The factors which determine the events are:

- the type of chemicals or hydrocarbons;
- the state; gas, liquid or solid;
- the processing conditions; pressure and temperature;
- the inventory or the amount of fuel which could be released;
- the causes of failure;
- the potential for escalation.

From this information, it is possible to identify and analyse the range of fires and explosions which might occur. It is relatively easy to determine the release rates of the fuels, the fire sizes, intensities, durations and the consequences for these events. Initial calculations are fit for purpose, say 70% accuracy, with more sophisticated tools available where greater refinement is needed. It is the predictability and limited range of these events which makes a hazard based approach to the management of fire and explosion hazards practicable.

While it may be easy to identify and analyse what might occur, the events are severe and potentially catastrophic. The initial event could be a flash fire, an explosion or a catastrophic rupture. This can cause injury and death to anyone working in the immediate area as was graphically demonstrated at Hickson and Welch (5).

An initial event may be a pool or jet fire which may engulf adjacent plant. It may continue at the same severity until escalation occurs. Recent work has shown that temperatures in excess of $1300^{\circ}C$ (6), heat fluxes over $350kw/m^2$ and explosion over-pressures of over 4 bar can occur in many plants processing simple hydrocarbons. Much more extreme effects might be experienced with other chemicals such as oxidising agents or explosive materials.

One characteristic of these events is the clearly defined increase in severity as failures occur. Unlike, for example, a forest fire which progressively spreads, sudden escalation can occur. This may be caused by a structural failure leading to the release of other fuels, ignition of large storage tanks or the catastrophic rupture of processing vessels. These escalating events can lead to further fatalities, both inside and beyond the plant and to major capital loss. While it might be possible to control smaller fires, often the escalating event is impossible to contain or extinguish and evacuation is the only option. By their nature, and open location, it is not practical to extinguish many hydrocarbon fires, particularly if they are gas jets, pressurised liquids, liquefied gases or oxidising agents. Therefore it may be necessary to let them burn out with protection systems provided to prevent escalation.

3.   **THE EVOLUTION OF THE INDUSTRY**

The industry is evolving and every time there is a mistake something will change and improve; from the details of codes and standards to a total revolution in our approach to hazard management. Different parts of the world are at different stages in the evolution process and the UK and Europe are at the forefront.

The industry has gone through three phases:

3.1   Managing Safety Systems

For many years, the culture and legislation was based on prescription and compliance; meeting the requirements of a series of design standards, codes and rules for prevention and protection systems. Each was written and evolved independently and, in most cases, they were adequate for most of the fire hazards. Their greatest fault is that they said what to do but not why. As a result, it was not possible to identify when the limits of applicability were exceeded. However, they did give a perfect defence; "we obeyed the rules." The chemical and onshore hydrocarbon industries changed to self regulation in the 1980s under the influence of the Control of Industrial Major Hazards Regulations (CIMAH) (7) but the offshore industry kept to the old course for a number of reasons - too many to discuss in this paper.

Piper Alpha was the last disaster where compliance with the rules was potentially inadequate. Nothing in the legislation required explosions to be considered at all and the fire protection systems were unsuitable for the types and severity of the fires. Possibly the most severe criticism is that most people in the industry did not recognise explosions as a threat. They did not conceive that an oil process fire could give flames extending 30-40m beyond the source module with toxic smoke engulfing the accommodation. Most people had no concept of the catastrophic consequences of a failed gas riser. As a result neither the people, nor the platform safety systems were prepared for the event.

3.2 Making a Case for Safety

Following Flixborough and Piper Alpha, the legislation changed both on and offshore, obliging the operators to prepare a Safety Case. These are either the CIMAH (7), soon to become COMAH (Control of Major Accident Hazards) (8) or Offshore Installation (Safety Case) Regulations (9). These require the analysis of major accident hazards, their likelihood and consequences, and an assessment of the risks to life both within and beyond the plant. These are assessed against criteria to judge if the risks are tolerable and "as low as reasonably practical". In this last concept, operators are required to examine any risk reducing measure to determine if it is economically viable by judging its contribution to saving life against the cost.

In principle, this approach is excellent as it requires all hazards to be addressed and there is no hiding behind a rule book which may not be applicable or appropriate. In theory, it gives the duty holders total freedom but it also gives them total responsibility. In practice, it has not achieved its full potential. The preparation of the Safety Case is an expensive and complicated process requiring input from specialist analysts. This is particularly noticeable where external consultants are used for the analysis of fire and explosion characteristics and for the numerical quantification of risk. This complex nature of the preparation of the Safety Case has made it a discrete and retrospective activity. In other words it has become separated from the day to day activities of individual designers and operators and it assesses a completed design rather than influencing it. The Safety Case can become a document for presentation to the authorities rather than a reference document for those with responsibilities for hazard management.

3.3 Integrated Hazard Management

In the offshore industry, the issue and implementation of the primary Safety Case Regulations (SCR) were followed by two other sets of secondary regulations, covering; Design and Construction (DCR) (10), and Prevention of Fires and Explosions, and Emergency Response (PFEER) (11). These support, and depend on the Safety Case. They were recommended by Lord Cullen "to give the Safety Case regime a solidity which it might otherwise lack". The time period between the primary and secondary regulations gave both the industry and the HSE the opportunity to look back at the initial implementation of the Safety Case legislation and to rectify any perceived deficiencies. The development of PFEER was one of positive co-operation between the regulator and industry. Both sides entered discussions with a common goal; to write regulations and guidance which would make a real contribution to reducing risks. The HSE prepared high quality, goal setting regulations while the United Kingdom Offshore Operators Association (UKOOA) wrote detailed guidance (12) to support them.

The subtle changes in regulations reflected a subtle shift in attitude from "prove its safe" to "understand the hazards and make it safe". This is a change from a retrospective analysis and rectification, to a proactive culture where everyone understands the hazards and tries to design and operate a safe plant so that it will not leak or catch fire. This new culture is slowly spreading through the industry. It is not in place everywhere but both the culture and the process, described in the next chapter, are advocated for other industries.

                                        C537/010 © IMechE 1997

4. THE PROCESS

The process starts with the culture. There needs to be an underlying desire by everyone, from plant and project managers down to individual designers and plant operators, to identify and understand the hazards and to reduce the risks from them. A compliance culture which seeks to fulfil the minutiae of regulations, codes and standards is wrong, as is a regulatory regime which promotes such compliance. With the correct culture, it is possible to create a proactive process which eliminates or minimises hazards at source rather than attempting to deal with potential or actual fires and explosions retrospectively. The process is simple and is described in the UKOOA Guidelines to the Management of Fire and Explosion Hazards (12). It is based on the six steps of a fire and explosion assessment (see Figure 1).

4.1 What can leak?

If hazards can be identified at an early stage in the conceptual design process or when an operational task is being planned, it may be possible to find a different and safer approach. This is the application of inherent safety and may either eliminate, or reduce the severity and consequences of the event.

4.2 How can it leak?

If every cause is identified; for example, corrosion, over-pressure, isolation failure etc., then each one can be addressed. This can minimise not only the likelihood but the size of the release; i.e. prevention.

4.3 What is the fire or explosion like?

In assessing the size, severity, location and duration of a fire or explosion, the most severe hazards can be identified. The factors which contribute to these characteristics are; the amount of fuel which might be released, the speed of detection, the rate of release, the size of the bunds into which liquids may be spilt, etc. This allows detection, shutdown, depressurisation and drainage systems to be optimised to reduce the severity of the event. In the case of explosion and unignited releases, it is also possible to minimise the chance of ignition and the overpressure by optimising the ventilation and layout. This is the control of the hazard.

4.4 What are the consequences?

Who would die in the initial and escalating event? What would be damaged by the explosion? What would be engulfed in flames for long enough to cause failure? The answers would allow the plant and operating philosophy to be optimised to reduce the exposure. Where this is not practical, appropriate protection systems can be applied to protect people, prevent failure or extinguish the fires; that is mitigation of the effects.

4.5 How can it escalate?

There will be a wide range of initial events throughout a plant and each one may have the potential for increasingly severe escalation as larger inventories are released and catch fire. The knowledge of both the likelihood of the initial event and the practicality of controlling the escalating event enables a decision to be taken on where to break the chain of events. The choices are:

- to invest only in prevention and to accept the consequences;
- to optimise the prevention and to provide protection against smaller events thereby preventing escalation;
- or to plan for the large or catastrophic event and to provide the resources to counteract it.

This is the selection of the strategies for each hazard and it will determine the whole site philosophy for fire and explosion hazard management.

4.6   What is the risk?

Each of the preceding five questions will progressively build a total picture of the numbers of people who might be killed, the cost of the damage and lost production, the potential public outrage and the likelihood of these consequences. This will take into account the frequency of the initial events and the probability that the safety systems will work and control the escalation. In the UK, these risks must be assessed and they must be reduced at least to minimum criteria and lower if practical. It is the question; "how good is good enough?" The results can be used to decide if prevention measures need to be improved or protection systems need to be more effective or reliable; for example the decision between fitting a fixed protection system or relying on manual response. This is the determination of the system quality.

The process will work if the answers to these questions are seen as basic design information and provided in time. It is better to have information of moderate quality which is available in time to help to get the design right, than to have the ultimate analysis which is delivered at the end of a project which identifies deficiencies and requires costly changes or improvements. The information should be collated and presented as a users guide to the hazards, remembering that designers need the information as well as plant operators. The documents are variously referred to as Hazard Registers, Hazard Management Plans or Hazard Analyses. Whatever the name, the concept is still the same. A plant in which the hazards are well understood and effectively managed is an order of magnitude safer than one which is operated in ignorance.

This may give the impression that the whole plant is analysed to the nth degree and that everything is designed from scratch. This is not the case. It is acceptable to take a standardised approach using recognised codes and standards for fire hazards which are well understood. However, it is essential that the appropriateness of the code for the particular hazard is verified. When specifying prevention measures, recognised codes, standards and procedural controls should be used, with Hazard and Operability Study (HAZOP) techniques to verify that these are suitable and effective. For control measures, the provision of equipment specified in accepted codes and standards is a good start point but it can be optimised to further reduce the hazard severity. In most cases, protection (mitigation) measures for major hazards will need to be based on an analysis of the hazards. There are few codes which could provide adequate protection against the wide range of hazards which might be encountered. If they did, they would probably grossly overprotect most areas and would be uneconomic.

Having decided how to manage each hazard and specified all of the safety systems, it is necessary to make sure that the equipment and people meet their intended performance throughout the life cycle of the plant. This covers detail design, construction, commissioning and operation. Systems must be testable and tested, and people must be competent and audited.

5.   MANAGING CHANGES

The previous sections discussed the design of the process, the assessment of the potential fires and explosions, the optimisation of the prevention and the provision of protection against smaller events, thereby preventing escalation. It is quite appropriate that these were treated in some detail as it has already been noted that the chemical and hydrocarbon industries operate in "steady state". Occasionally the process is not in "steady state", when there is a need to make a process change or to carry out maintenance or inspections. These situations have to be managed using a similar approach:

What can occur?
How can it occur?
What is the fire/explosion potential?
What are the consequences?
How can it escalate?
What is the risk?

5.1   Management of Change

In the case of a process change, the extremes of the operating envelope will already have been examined in the HAZOP Study technique. Occasionally changes to the process, hardware and operating parameters may be required to optimise the process further or a new pump may be required to replace an old unit. These changes are handled by a "Management of Change" where the six questions are analysed by a small team of experienced engineers. In many cases the analysis may only take a few hours, but for larger changes this make take a few days. An increase in throughput may increase the erosion inside the piping, so leading to loss of wall thickness and process fluid leakage leading to a potential fire. Increase in velocity may also cause piping and plant to resonate leading to metal fatigue and process fluid leakage. An increase in the process temperature may increase corrosion rates or may create adverse by-product reactions, which in turn lead to a potential risk of explosion. A new pump may have different characteristics which may violate the design intent. This is very often ignored, to the jeopardy of safety - there is a rule of "like for like".

The "Management of Change" may appear to be pedantic but the lack of management of change is one of the major precursors to incidents, as exemplified by Flixborough (1) and, to a lesser extent, Piper Alpha (4).

5.2 Management of Maintenance

It is inevitable that equipment will break down in service (wear out) and require overhaul. Such maintenance inevitably means isolation and removal in a safe manner. The control of this work is carried out by a "Permit to Work" (PTW) in which the six questions indicated are addressed:

What is to be done?
What can occur or go wrong?
What is the potential?
What are the consequences?
How can it escalate, and what controls must be put in place to prevent the event occurring, or to recover from the event?
What is the final risk and can it be done in a better way (the inherently safer way)?

The PTW may be generated by a Task Risk Assessment. This is a very powerful tool as it involves both the supervisors and those who will carry out the work. The output is documented in the PTW but the involvement of the operators ensures that they understand the hazard and endorse the precautions.

Each maintenance task will be reviewed in detail and the controls clearly specified in the PTW before the work is carried out. The conditions for the work will be verified by a local visit and a discussion between the owner (operations) and the maintenance team, so that there can be no doubt or confusion by either party as to what is to be done and how it is to be done.

Where activities are planned which clearly increase the chance of an incident occurring or its consequences, closer examination is needed to decide if it is safe to proceed at all. If it does proceed, strict precautions and safeguards will be implemented. In the case of welding, for example, all flammable materials would be removed or covered with fire blankets, portable gas detectors would monitor the working area, and the site would be subject to routine inspection or continuous observation.

By managing change from the previously safe, steady state condition, the potential for fires and explosions can be reduced to as low as is reasonably practicable. Once again, these systems must be executed by competent people and audited.

6. THE PETROCHEMICAL AND OFFSHORE INDUSTRY IN 1997

The preceding text outlined an evolving process. The industry has not fully embraced and implemented the process in Section 4. In most cases, they have to live with what they have in terms of plant layout, design standards and equipment provision. In new designs, the principles in Section 4 are acknowledged and endorsed but most projects are now fast track and, in many cases, the results of the analysis are still arriving too late to have a significant effect on the design.

The two areas which are improving are the culture and the understanding of hazards. All new plants are being designed in the knowledge of the hazards and effective systems are in place to prevent and control them. Existing plants are developing hazard descriptions (Fig. 2) and hazard management plans (Fig. 3). As a result both operators and emergency response personnel have a much better idea of the fire and explosion hazards on the plant.

One area where progress still needs to be made is in the perception of what constitutes a safe plant. There is still a belief among many people that blast resistant fire-walls, fire-pumps, deluge systems, extensive detection and passive protection are the critical features. These are secondary. The safe plant is one which does not leak. It is safe because it is well designed, well built and operated properly within its limits by competent people. Prevention is better than cure. This must be encouraged by regulations and endorsed by everyone; operators, design contractors and the HSE inspectors.

References

1. Parker, R.J., The Flixborough Disaster - Report of the Court of Inquiry, 1975. HMSO, London.
2. Pietersen, C.M., Analysis of the LPG Incident in San Juan Ixhuatepec, Mexico City, 19/1/84 - TNO, The Hague, Netherlands.
3. Various Press Reports. Los Alfraques
4. Lord Cullen, The Report into the Piper Alpha Disaster. 1990, HMSO, London.
5. The Investigation into the fire at Hickson and Welch. 1994, HSE Books.
6. The Joint Industry Project on Fire and Explosion; details from the Steel Construction Institute
7. Control of Major Accident Regulations. S1 1984, No. 1902.
8. COMAH (being developed)
9. Offshore Installations; Safety Case, Regulations, S1 1992, No. 2885.
10. Offshore Installations and Wells (Design and Construction) Regulations, SI 1996, No. 913
11. Prevention of Fire and Explosions, and Emergency Response on Offshore Installations; Approved Code of Practice and Guidance, ISBN 0-7176-0874-3
12. Guidelines on the Management of Fire and Explosion published by UKOOA

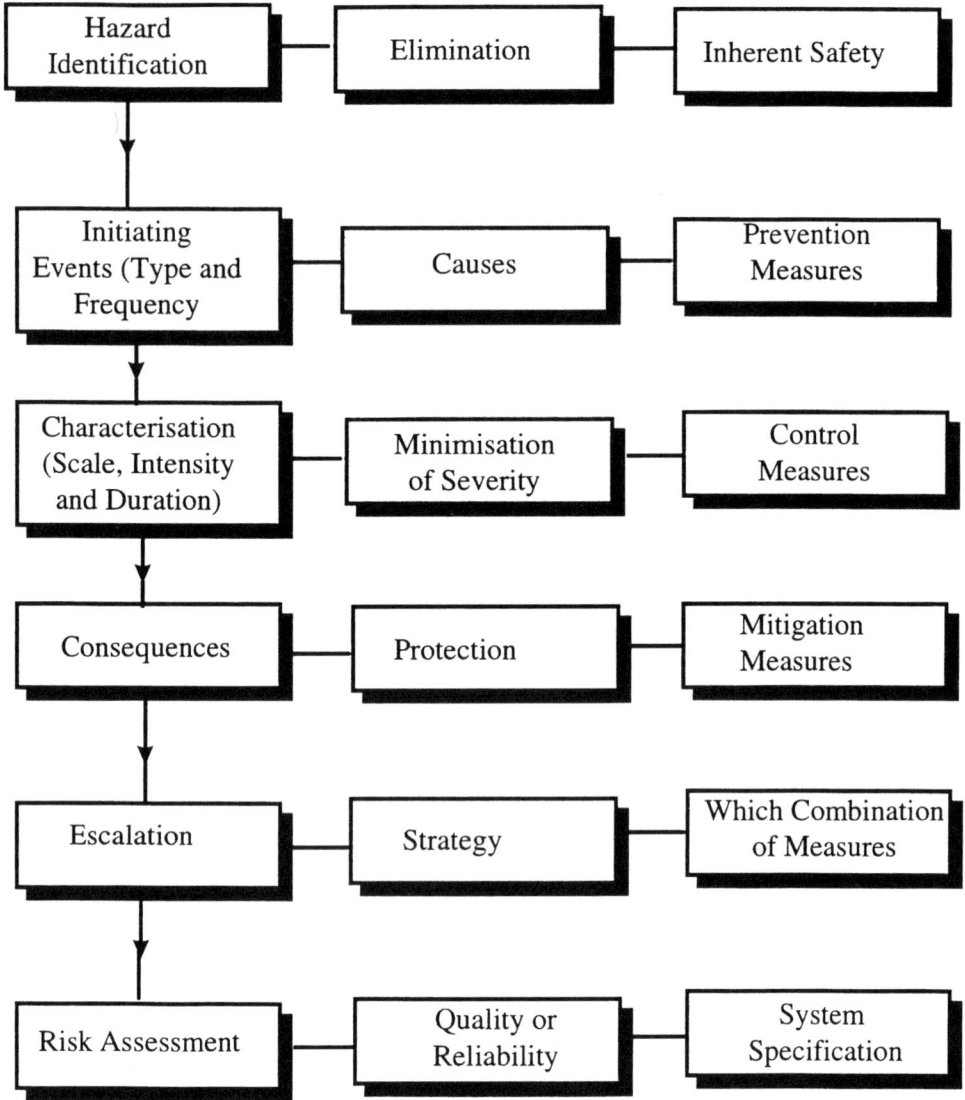

Figure 1

Fire hazard analysis and management

FIRE CASE FOR   SEPARATOR OIL FIRE

INVENTORY SYSTEM/EQUIPMENT	PROBABLE FIRE TYPE
Separator V-1002A, Desalter/Dehydrator V1-1003A and associated pipework	Pool Fire

FIRE CHARACTERISTICS

Ignition may be preceded by an oil release giving up to 25mm oil depth in the bunded area. Ignition would give a pool fire from the point of release.

The pool fire would cover the bunded area with flames to a height of 15-25m (associated with large quantities of smoke). Heat fluxes and temperatures would be 1100°C and 200kW/m² for pool fires. The oil spill would drain to the outer gully

FIRE SIZE	FIRE SIZE	FIRE SIZE	ASSUMED ESCALATION TIMES
Oil Release through 10mm	Oil Release through 25mm	Oil Release through 50mm	10 mins (adjacent train)
Pre-ESD: 0.75kg/s released and burns as a pool fire in an equivalent pool area of 18.75m² either (a) inside the bund area or (b) outside the bund area.	Pre-ESD: 4.7kg/s released and burns as a pool fire in an equivalent pool area of 117.5m² in the same ways as the 10mm case either (a) inside the bund area or (b) outside the bund area.	Pre-ESD: 18.8kg/s released and burns as a pool fire in an equivalent pool area of 470m2 of the bund or outside the bund area.	
Equivalent pool diameter - 4.9m. Flame height = 5.2m. Total fire duration = 34 hrs.	Equivalent pool diameter = 12.2m Flame height = 9.9m. Total Fire duration = 5hrs 28mins.	Equivalent pool diameter = 24.4m. Flame height = 24.2m Total fire duration = 1hr 24mins	

ESCALATION DAMAGE CONSEQUENCES

In the event of a pool fire around the separators, the following may be involved and create escalation:

The Inventory from the adjacent separation train.

Dump Tank T-1001 may be exposed but would be unlikely to fail because of insulation. Piperacks are not passively protected and some escalation may occur if the supports fail and the oil lines may release their contents

ASSUMPTIONS

1. Bund disposes of all pre-released oil except for 25mm layer.
2. The drains only dispose of any oil in excess of a release rate of 9.4kg/s following ESD
3. ESD occurs in 3 mins.
4. Isolated inventory released consists of the contents of 1 separation train and the interconnecting pipework to the pumps.

COMMENTS

Fire should not spill into next bund as each bund slopes away from the separator thereby forcing the fire to collect and burn in a smaller area away from the separators.

Fig 2: An example of a simple fire description for an onshore plant

© IMechE 1997 C537/010

FIRE HAZARD MANAGEMENT PLANT FOR			SEPARATORS	
METHODS	IMPORTANCE	REFERENCE	RESPONSIBLE POSITION	COMMENTS
PREVENTION Overpressurisation protection PSV 10646 A/B & 10651 A/B	Medium	Maintenance Procedures Terminal Planned Maintenance Programme	Maintenance Supervisor	Overpressure unlikely.
Corrosion protection Control of activities in area	High High	Company & Industry Standards Terminal Emergency Plan Terminal Competency Scheme	Maintenance Supervisor Process Supervisor	
DETECTION & ALARM CCTV	High	Vendor Maintenance Procedures Vendor Maintenance Programme	CCR Operator	
Bunds and drains	High	Terminal Operating Procedures Terminal Competency Scheme	Plant Operator	Pay particular attention to ensure drains are open and clear.
Isolation Valves: ESV 10901	High	Terminal Operating Procedures	Maintenance Supervisor	
MITIGATION/RESPONSE Hydrofoam monitors	Medium	Terminal Planned Maintenance Programme Terminal Competency Scheme	Safety Officer	See Emergency Response Plan

Fig 3 - An Example of a Hazard Management Plan

C537/011/97

Hazards and their management

G-C CHAZOT
Eurotunnel

1. INTRODUCTION

Safety of passengers and staff is a paramount objective within Eurotunnel. In order to achieve this, we have developed a comprehensive safety strategy based on:-

- planning out hazards at the design stage;

- applying operating procedures which avoid hazards;

- as a result, keeping hazards as low as reasonably practicable (ALARP);

- minimising the consequences of any undesirable event without delay;

- development of emergency responses to contain and deal with any incident.

2. DESIGN AND CONSTRUCTION

From the early days of the project, safety and the avoidance of hazards were foremost in the minds of the design, construction and commissioning teams. The following are examples of this approach.

The Tunnels
- Separate running tunnels for the two rail tracks:
  - apart from periods of single line working for maintenance purposes etc., these tunnels are uni-directional
  - risk of head-on collision virtually eliminated;
  - no hazard from vandalism or extreme weather;

- Central Service Tunnel between two rail tunnels (cost £1 billion):
  - provides access for electronically guided rubber tyred maintenance vehicles and emergency services;
  - 'safe haven' for passengers and staff in the event of an evacuation
  - runs full length of tunnel complex and connects every 342.9 metres to rail tunnels via cross passage doors.

- Continuous walkways on both sides of each rail track:
  - in the event of a derailment, trains would remain upright and in line;
  - walkway on side of Service Tunnel facilitates evacuation from trains.

- 2 ventilation systems:
  - plant at both ends of tunnel with high degree or redundancy;
- Normal Ventilation System
  - air passes through Service Tunnel and into rail tunnels through non-returnable vents;
  - air pressure in Service Tunnel always higher than in rail tunnels, thus reinforcing concept of the Service Tunnel as a 'safe haven' i.e. no possibility of smoke from rail tunnels penetrating Service Tunnel.

- Supplementary Ventilation System:
  - used only in rail tunnels;
  - can blow/extract air in either direction;
  - main purpose is control of smoke to assist evacuation and fire-fighting.

- 2 sources of power supply:
  - electricity fed from both UK/French power grids during normal operations;
  - either is capable of keeping trains moving throughout tunnel complex;
  - if both go down, standby diesel generators which can provide essential services e.g. lighting and communications.

- Continuous firemain through Service Tunnel:
  - outlets every 125 m in both running tunnels for water for fire hoses.

- Many other examples within the tunnels:
  - fire detectors which can detect flame, smoke and CO levels, every 1½-2½ kms;
  - hot wheel bearing/dragging equipment detectors;
  - tunnel linings made from some of the strongest concrete in the world.

but same principle was applied to the design and construction of rolling stock.

Shuttle Trains

Tourist Shuttles

- each carrier wagon has a series of detectors which can detect hydrocarbon vapours, flame and smoke;

- video cameras which are automatically operational if a detector is activated or a passenger presses a call button to the Chef de Train (Train Captain) A series of pictures from the wagon concerned is immediately displayed on the Chef de Train's console.

- apart from hand held extinguishers there are:

  · AFFF (Aqueous Film Forming Foam) which immediately covers any fuel spillage from a vehicle which has drained into a specially built holding tank;

- Halon 1301 which can be automatically released, but only if the environment in the wagon was life threatening (extensive programme of evacuation exercises has shown that the chances of release before evacuation from the wagon is complete is remote).

- Shuttle wagons are built to contain a fire for up to 30 minutes:

- passengers evacuate longitudinally into adjacent wagons and shuttle continues its journey;

  · shuttle proceeds to special emergency sidings (in both terminals) where facilities are available for fire-fighters to deal with the situation.

- As far as practicable, wagons built with fire resistant materials:-

  · avoids smoke/toxic fumes when heated.

HGV Shuttles

- totally different concept: drivers are segregated from their vehicles and travel in a Club-Car;
- however, there is a fire detection system on each loader wagon, which if activated, will register on the Chef de Train's console which is in the Club-Car.

Locomotives

A common cause of collisions on railways is driver error; however, all electric locomotives used in the Channel tunnel are fitted with ATP (Automatic Train Protection) which guards against this.

The signalling system ensures that the speed at which the locomotive should be travelling is displayed in the cab. If a driver does not observe this and ignores warnings, the ATP system takes over and can bring the train to a stop.

Two Locomotives on each train

- on all Tourist/HGV shuttles and Eurostars, there is a locomotive at each end;

- one loco. is capable of ensuring that the shuttle/train concerned can exit the tunnel should the other loco fail.
- provides capability, in the event of an incident, to reverse train movement with loco and driver at the head.

3. SELECTION OF STAFF

What has been outlined gives, I trust, a strong flavour of the immense activity which was undertaken to avoid hazards as the project moved forward. However, at the same time, we were mounting a heavy recruitment programme and it was essential that we selected people of good calibre, with the right personal qualities and attitudes, particularly towards customer service and safety. This was a very time consuming process, but the result was worthwhile. Remember, we had not started commercial operations, so we could claim no safety culture, which stems largely from experience over a period of time. Having people onboard, however, who were committed to safety and understood that every employee is responsible for safety of operations under his/her control, helped to compensate for our "adolescence" as an organisation at that time.

4. SAFETY DOCUMENTATION

We recruited people from a wide range of transport undertakings eg. BR/SNCF/London Underground/Docklands Light Railway/Lille Metro/the Ferries;

In preparing our safety documentation, we drew on their experience, with help from outside specialists, reflecting where appropriate, "best practices";

This documentation is divided into three separate but interlinked sections:

Level 1	Safety Arrangements
Level 2	Operating Principles
Level 3	Operating Instructions

The Level 1 documents set down the general safety rules which cover the whole Eurotunnel system of transportation, while Level 2 contains the principles which support the rules. Level 3 sets out the detailed operating instructions covering every task which is undertaken.

Throughout the preparation of this documentation, avoidance of hazards was again a major consideration. The following are examples of this approach during the preparation of operating instructions:

HGV Shuttles

Although research suggested that HGV parking brakes were adequate to hold vehicles if there was a sharp brake application by the locomotive during rail transit, we believed that the risk of vehicle movement, however unlikely, was unacceptable because of the possible implications;

As a result, all lorries are chocked while in rail transit. At present up to 8 chocks are applied manually to each vehicle. This is a very expensive process and the search continues for an automatic system of vehicle restraint.

Tourist Shuttles

The biggest potential hazard on tourist shuttles is a fuel fire, so our attention focused on procedures to be followed by our customers:

- no smoking,
- hand brake on,
- vehicle in 1st gear or "Parking",
- no blocking of walkways,
- vehicles parked close to each other,
- no refuelling or vehicle repairs during rail transit

I would add that in the event that there is an incident onboard a tourist shuttle, we have a 3 stage response, again designed to manage hazards appropriately i.e.:

- Level 1 alarm

  caused by the activation of any one detector or a customer pushing the call button   to the Chef de Train. A member of Eurotunnel's patrolling staff would go to the wagon concerned to investigate;

- Level 2 alarm

  caused by the activation of any two detectors in a wagon. There would be an immediate evacuation of passengers into adjacent wagons;

- Level 3 alarm

  probably caused by a rapid growth fire,

  automatic release of Halon, but system designed so that this takes place as late as possible to ensure maximum time is available for evacuation.

5. MINIMUM OPERATING REQUIREMENTS

Because of the complexity of our system, we also developed a series of Minimum Operating Requirements (MORs) which set down the boundaries of the safe operating envelope for rolling stock, each sub-system of fixed equipment, and staff involved in transport system safety. These MORs were established for:-

- normal operating status,
- minimum requirements for normal commercial service,
- degraded operating modes which were acceptable and still within the boundaries of safe operation (in many cases, for a given period of time only).

A simple example is the list of the requirements in respect of local Fire Detection Units; LFDUs which are located in the cross passages between the Service Tunnel and the railway tunnels, monitor the fire detection stations in the railway tunnels and sensors in the technical rooms:

- normal operating status   - all LFDU's are operational
- minimum requirements for   - not more than one LFDU inoperative
- commercial service
- degraded mode   - two to five LFDU's inoperable;
                                     closure after 30 days of both running
                                     tunnels if not operable by that time
                                   - over five LFDUs inoperative;
                                     immediate closure of both tunnels.

- these MORs were established on the basis of detailed risk analysis, and conformance with them is monitored round the clock in our Railway Control Centre (RCC). They are a vital tool for the management of safety and take away the risk of making hasty judgements in difficult situations which could be fatal.

6. SAFETY CASE

By agreement with the Channel Tunnel Safety Authority, and as a fundamental part of the risk management process, Eurotunnel prepared a Safety Case in 1994 prior to start up of commercial operations, and this was published in June of that year. The preparation of a safety case is well known for nuclear power stations and offshore oil and gas installations, but Eurotunnel's was the first on any comparable scale in the world of surface transport.

Eurotunnel's Safety Case was based on how the system was expected to operate taking account of its design, procedures and training of staff, and reflected forecast traffic volumes for the year 1996. It deals with the system description, design safety principles, risk criteria, normal and emergency operations, qualitative and quantitative risk assessment and a description of the safety management systems used by Eurotunnel. This detailed document demonstrated that residual risks were low and that there were no further measures which could reasonably be taken to lower the risk level even more. Further, the Safety Case demonstrated that risks in the Channel Tunnel system, were approximately 20 times less than those observed at that time on the UK and French railway networks.

Under the Railways (Safety Case) Regulations 1994, our Safety Case has to be revised every 3 years and we are currently completing this process. We have taken traffic forecasts for the year 2000 as the basis of this revision, as traffic volumes have risen steadily and, of course, we have the benefit of 3 years of invaluable experience behind us - including the many lessons learnt from the fire which we had in the tunnel on Monday   18 November 1996.

I would stress that our Safety Case is treated internally as a living document. Any proposed modifications to equipment or rolling stock, or methods of working must, before being progressed, first be tested against the stated risk criteria contained in the Safety Case, to ensure that there is no reduction in the overall level of safety.

Eurotunnel's Safety Case revision is being undertaken against the background of Eurotunnel's responsibilities as an operator. Under the Railway (Safety Case) Regulations 1994, Eurotunnel also has the responsibility as an infrastructure provider, to scrutinise and accept safety cases of other operators providing services through the tunnel. Eurotunnel, before accepting any such safety case, must satisfy itself that the other operator is meeting the standards Eurotunnel has laid down in its own Safety Case.

7. MANAGEMENT OF SAFETY

Responsibility for overseeing and monitoring of safety performance throughout the Company is vested in the Director, Health, Safety & Quality. As shown in Figure 1 below, he reports direct to the Group Managing Director who is responsible to the Joint Board for the safe management of the Company's activities, and therefore stands independent of all other Directors and Departments. He also has access, if necessary, to the Chairman of the Joint Board Safety Committee.

Figure 1

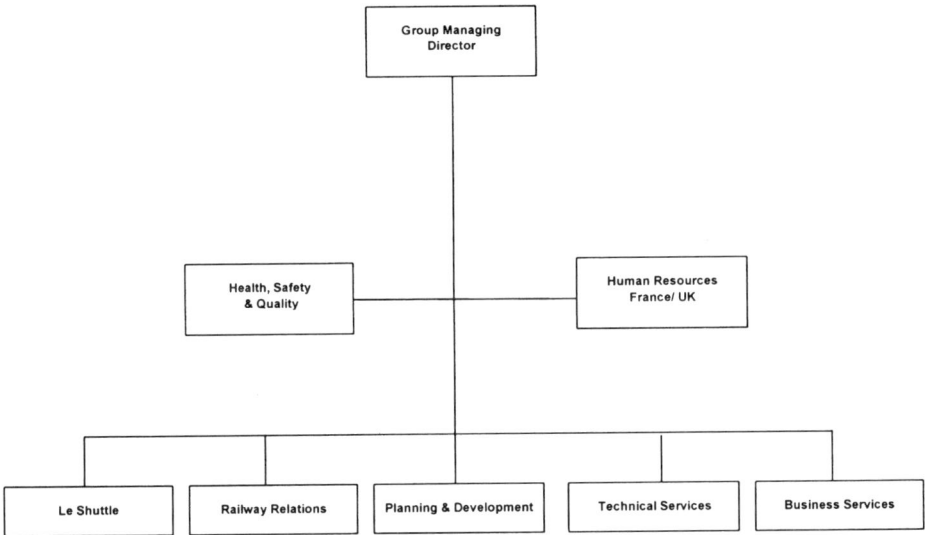

The Joint Board Safety Committee (see Figure 2 below) has been organised to combine board level authority with independence of outlook. It consists of executive and non-executive Directors, including the Chairman and Group Managing Director, but is chaired by a non-executive Director. The Director, Health, Safety & Quality, attends all meetings of this Committee which are held bi-monthly.

Below the Joint Board Safety Committee, the main forum for discussion of safety issues and resolution of problems, is the Operations Safety Committee, which meets monthly. The Director, HSQ is one of the Co-Chairmen of this Committee, which consists of all Departmental and other senior line managers involved in the operation and maintenance of our system. The Committee is supported by a Rules and Regulations Committee, to which all proposals for changes to operating principles and instructions must be submitted.

Each Departmental Manager, in turn, holds regular meetings with this/her management team, at which safety is high on the agenda. These teams include Safety and Quality Correspondents who assist the Departmental Managers in meeting their obligations to ensure that all staff are adequately trained, and are conversant with, and abide by, all company and legislative Health and Safety rules. Although S&Q Correspondents work for line managers, they have a strong 'dotted line' relationship with the HSQ Directorate, and meet monthly under the chairmanship of the Deputy Director, Health, Safety and Quality.

In addition to the above Committee structure, which consists of staff appointed by management, there is a Health & Safety Committee in the UK, which apart from the Chairman who is the Director, HS&Q, consists of representatives elected by the staff. There is an equivalent Committee on the French side called the Comité d'Hygiène de Sécurité et des Conditions de Travail (CHSCT);

I would stress at this point that primary responsibility for safety rests with line managers, i.e. ownership of safety is in the line and all levels of management and supervisory staff have four common major responsibilities for which they will be held accountable:

- to intervene and cease any operation which is patently unsafe,
- to ensure that safe working practices in their areas exist are clearly defined and formally documented in current official texts,
- to ensure that those practices are implemented on an ongoing basis,
- to monitor the degree of compliance with and effectiveness of Eurotunnel's safety standards.

It is Eurotunnel's commitment that managers who have responsibility for safety of equipment and processes, also have the resources to fulfil their obligations;

One of the means by which line management fulfils the above responsibilities, is Safety Briefings. Following a serious incident or accident, it is frequently the case that such talks are held in order to learn from experience and improve safety in the future. Within Eurotunnel, this is known as 'Retour d'Expérience (REX)'.

Figure 2

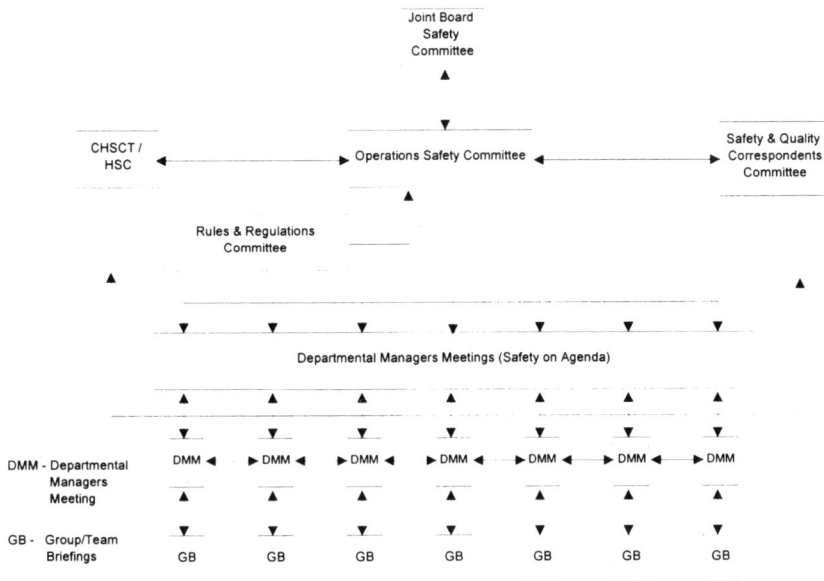

8. SAFETY MANAGEMENT SYSTEMS

"En Garde" System

The "En Garde" system is perhaps the most single important tool within Eurotunnel for monitoring safety. It is a system which allows recording of both accidents and incidents. An accident is defined as an undesirable event which causes either injury to a person, damage to property or loss to process. An incident is defined as an undesirable event which under slightly different circumstances, could have caused injury to a person, damage to property or loss to process. The "En Garde" system records not only the facts of the event, but also codes it with both the actual severity, the potential severity and the likelihood of recurrence from which the actual loss and the potential risk of the vent can be calculated. This enables Eurotunnel to categorise events into the ones that had potentially the most serious consequences, and to prioritise correct actions to deal with these events. It also has a system of key wording which allows different attributes to be given to particular events such that sorting them can be done to bring out trends and common features that otherwise might not be apparent. Detailed analysis of the figures coming from "En Garde" enables Eurotunnel to make decisions and implement strategies that proactively reduce the risk to both passengers and staff on the system as well as the potential loss to the Company. It also provides a means of monitoring the actual process of dealing with accidents and incidents from the initial recording of the facts through their analysis, the making of recommendations, the implementation of the actions, the verification that the actions taken have resolved the problem and the feedback to staff that the incident has been closed.

I would emphasise that the cornerstone of the success of "En Garde" lies in Eurotunnel's philosophy of where no employee will be formally disciplined if they report unintentional errors what they have made or that they observe in any part of the Company operation. A distinction is drawn between unintentional errors or mistakes and gross misconduct, since the latter will attract disciplinary measures appropriate to that misdeed. This philosophy has been endorsed at the highest level of Eurotunnel and is adopted by employees at all levels.

This culture is founded on the principle that knowledge of accidents and incidents is vital to Eurotunnel's well-being from a health and safety point of view, and that unless an open and trusting cultures is employed, this knowledge will not be forthcoming. Repetition of the same error or mistake will not necessarily be viewed in the same light.

There have been a number of examples of "En Garde" assisting in identifying trends, but perhaps the most interesting, related to fire barrier protection devices onboard Tourist Shuttles. These were retractable arms built into the floor of wagons, which when raised, protected vehicles from rolling forwards or backwards into the fire barrier at the ends of each wagon. However, reporting through "En Garde" identified that when these arms were folded down, there were a considerable number of cases of damage occurring to the underframe of cars during the loading/unloading process, and this presented a major fire hazard. In conjunction with outside specialists and following considerable research, we developed energy absorbing blocks which we were able to mount on the wagon pass doors. These were as effective as the restraining devices in ensuring that a rolling vehicle did not damage the fire barriers, but the removal of the devices not only stopped any further damage to vehicles, but also eliminated a hazard which presented the risk of trips and falls by passengers.

Loss Control/Risk Assessment
A pilot Loss Control system which was a modification to 'En Garde' was recently introduced, and will shortly be reviewed. At the same time, we have successfully developed 'in house', a software package to assist line management in the preparation of risk assessments. When fully developed, these two additional systems will add considerably to the armoury available to handle hazards.

Safety Audits
Annually, we prepare a safety audit programme which is carried out by the Health, Safety and Quality Directorate. Until 1997, audits were based on a review by departments i.e. vertically, but we found as a result of these, that the areas requiring additional line management attention tended to be the same right across the organisation. Indeed, this was confirmed by the results of a Safety Questionnaire given to every member of staff last autumn. For this year, therefore, our safety audits are 'topic' based across the organisation as a whole i.e. they will be horizontal, and enable more time to be devoted to priority issues.

9. MANAGEMENT OF FIRE AND EXPLOSIONS

As this is the title of this Conference it is only appropriate that I should say something about the management of fire within Eurotunnel.

During the early stages of the commissioning of our systems, we established a series of Table Top Exercises designed to test the procedures we had prepared for handling serious incidents and accidents, including fire, particularly those involving evacuation and rescue in the tunnels. Eurotunnel and the Emergency Services (both UK and France) participated in these and a great deal was learnt, particularly in terms of co-ordination between the parties concerned. As commissioning progressed, a series of small evacuation exercises was undertaken by Eurotunnel in the tunnels, involving longitudinal evacuation through wagons in transit as well as from stationary trains.

Prior to the granting of Operating Certificates for Eurostar and tourist shuttle services, there were full evacuation exercises in the tunnels, each involving several hundred passengers. We also gave an undertaking to the Intergovernmental Commission to undertake each year a comprehensive Bi-National Exercise with Eurotunnel, the UK and French Emergency Services, and National Railways participating. The scenarii chosen for these exercises to date, have been based on serious accidents and the last such exercise on 9/10 November last year assumed an explosion in transit.

In addition, we have fortnightly exercises in the tunnel simulating tourist shuttle evacuations in conjunction with professional fire-fighters.

However, the first major test of our response to a serious fire was on 18 November 1996, when there was a fire onboard an HGV shuttle in the tunnel en route from France to the UK. You will know from what you have read in the press, heard on the radio or seen on television, that this fire was serious enough to close 1/6th of our rail tunnel system for 6 months, and suspension by Eurotunnel during that period of its HGV shuttle services pending a review and improvements to the safe operations of these trains.

A number of issues emerged from this accident:

- the equipment in the tunnels and rolling stock performed very largely in accordance with the design specifications,

- the global strategy for handling a fire of this kind as described in our Safety Case, had been correctly transposed to the procedures in place,

- our tiered approach to safety of passengers and staff was successful i.e:-

  · seek to exit the complete shuttle from the tunnel,
  · if unable to do this, carry out a controlled stop and detach locomotive and Club-Car and exit these,
  · if unable to do this, evacuate passengers and staff into the Service Tunnel

Procedures were for the most part correctly followed, the way in which the fire was managed showed that the operators concerned, faced with numerous and complex procedures, were not sufficiently trained in the management of emergency situations.

Since the fire, we have taken a number of important corrective actions to improve safety and when this process is complete, the number of actions completed will have exceeded 100. Improvements have been made to equipment, procedures have been simplified and amended to effect a quicker response, and all staff involved in the operation of HGV shuttle services have received 'top-up' refresher training in the handling of accidents and emergency situations.

There was nothing wrong with the basic training that these people received, but the accident proved that the number of exercises and simulations we had undertaken were insufficient and on the night we were 'caught on the wrong foot'. We have put this right and now work to the principle that we must have training, training and more training!

10.CONCLUSION

We are still a comparatively young Company and one which is still developing its safety culture, but much has been done to eliminate or manage hazards and this work will continue. The accident on 18 November last year really was a 'baptism of fire' for Eurotunnel, but we have come out of that experience as a more robust and mature organisation on which we can build for the future.

Despite the seriousness of the fire, no passenger or member of staff suffered serious physical injury. Some 16 million other passengers also travelled through the tunnel in 1996 without serious injury - an encouraging record.

© Eurotunnel

C537/012/97

Management of fire – retrofit

D COWARD GIFireE
London Underground Limited, UK

The Oxford Dictionary states:-
'Retrofit - to incorporate changes and developments introduced after completion.'
It is a word that is becoming common in the UK, but has been used in 'Fire Safety' in America for over 20 years.

In order to understand the need for this approach by London Underground Ltd when undertaking station improvements. we must consider the events of the night of November 18th 1987 and the Kings Cross fire.

At 19.29 hours that evening a fire was reported by a member of the public on escalator No 4. Unfortunately the fire rapidly engulfed the station ticket hall with the tragic result that 31 people died. (30 members of the public and 1 fire officer). This incident obviously aroused major public concern, and the Secretary of State for Transport on the 23rd November 1987, appointed Mr Desmond Fennel OBE, QC to undertake a formal investigation into the circumstances of the Kings Cross fire.

I do not intend to list all the team but four assessors were also appointed to assist him.

1. Professor Bernard Crossland - who had been President of the Institute of Mechanical Engineers 1986/7.

2. Sir Peter Darby who had been Her Majesty's Chief Inspector of Fire Services for England and Wales and prior to this was Chief Officer of the London Fire Brigade.

3. Major Anthony King - an Inspecting Officer of Railways in the Department of Transport's Railway Inspectorate and finally:-

4. Dr Alan Roberts - Director of the Explosions and Flame laboratory, the Health and Safety Executive, Buxton.

It is clear that the knowledge and diversity of the team allowed all aspects of the inquiry to be reviewed in depth.

The 'Fennell' report as it was to be known, was far reaching and the final document was presented to the Secretary of State for Transport on 21st October 1988. It was a hard hitting investigation and all parties involved in the incident received some criticism. In all, the final report made 157 recommendations through a range of topics from training to emergency services communication.

During the investigation it became obvious that the Fire Precaution Act 1971 as amended by the Health and Safety at Work Act 1971, was not clear with regards to sub-surface stations, and it was left with Counsel to resolve the legal interpretation, which after much debate stated that the legislation of the day did not cover Sub-surface Railway Stations.

The major problem was over the definition in the Act of a 'building' and it was concluded that a sub-surface station did not meet this definition. It was also evident that application of the 71 Act per-se would be unlikely to achieve the desired improvements to fire safety for two very good reasons. Firstly, a fire certificate is only required where more than 20 persons are employed to work on the premises or more that 10 elsewhere than on the ground floor. Very few stations would have qualified under these criteria. The second reason revolved around the work which would have been required to bring most underground stations to an acceptable standard in terms of escape routes. Not only would it have been prohibitively expensive but, in most cases, it would have been impossible to achieve because of the existing infrastructure on the surface above these stations. Much of the underground system in London would have closed for an indefinite period and, in all probability, some of it for ever.

The subsequent result of this was the implementation of The Fire Precautions (Sub-surface Railway Stations) Regulations 1989. These regulations were made under powers conferred on the Home Secretary under Section 12(1) of the Fire Precautions Act 1971 and came into force on the 18th September 1989.

The 'Regulations' were very prescriptive mainly for the reasons just detailed, and relevant sections were phased to become operative over three years. They were arranged under thirteen parts and for the purposes of this paper I will discuss the problems associated with :-

a)   Regulation 5: Means for fighting fire
b)   Regulation 6: Means for detecting fire and giving warning in case of fire
and
c)   Regulation 7: Fire resisting construction in premises

Whilst I will discuss other elements that created problems I do not intend to cover each section of the Regulations in detail.

It must be stressed that London Underground did not sit back to wait for the findings of the Fennell report and within days of the fire had :-

a)   Started reviewing the fire systems within the market place to provide automatic fire suppression under escalators (Regulation 5). Numerous tests and designs were reviewed by the then Electrical and Mechanical Engineer, and a specification produced for a hybrid system known as 'Escalator Sprinkler Protection System' (ESPS). It was eventually accepted by the 'business' and is now the agreed protection for London Underground escalators.

b)   Extended the existing 'Material Code of Practice' and endorsed it ay Board level as Corporate Policy. Under this code all materials used underground must satisfy certain criteria with regard to flammability and smoke/toxic fume emissions.

Management Dilemma

It was now decision time for LUL Management as they had to undertake actions from 'Fennell' and meet compliance with the 'Regulations' which at this time affected 115 stations. Did they close the network down as decided in Strathclyde or keep the stations open and retrofit every station?

London Underground stations are operational from approximately 05.00 through to the last train generally 00.30 which, as can be appreciated, only gives a limited time for contractors to undertake any work. This creates major problems as contractors cannot even begin to bring materials and plant into stations before the last train has passed through and, in general, storage on the station is not permitted, either by LULs own strict code or the requirements of the 'Regulations'.

Problems

The major problems faced bu LUL in carrying out a retrofit of fire systems on stations were:-

a)   Short Working Period
b)   Premium rates and paying for complete shift
c)   High volume of work
d)   Insufficient contractors available
e)   Inability to procure sufficient parts and equipment in the short term such as fire doors
f)   Abortive work where emergency track or operational requirements do not allow track power to be shut down.

However, after deliberation LUL Management decided to take the route of 'Retrofit' and, having made the decision, discussed the implications with the Regulatory Authorities ie HM Inspectors of Railways and LFCDA. Meetings took place to agree works required to be undertaken.
Because of the manner in which the 'Regulations' were enacted, every station was subjected to joint LUL/LFCDA inspection and schedules of interim works were produced prior to full compliance being achieved especially in respect of 'compartmentation' (Regulation 5).

Stations at that time did not have any manual or automatic fire warning systems (Regulation 6). To keep stations functioning management had to undertake a massive recruitment of staff who were employed literally as human fire detectors. Many were retired LUL staff and were given the unkind title by the media of 'Dads Army'.

Many rooms on stations throughout the system contained sensitive electrical equipment, much of it old but essential to maintaining an operational railway. These rooms, then and now, remain secured and only approved and trained staff are allowed to enter them. This added a further dimension to the problem because 'Dads Army' could not enter such rooms. It was therefore agreed that, as an interim arrangement, these rooms would be protected by stand-alone automatic fire detection systems. Over 1000 systems were installed consisting of a smoke detector and control panel inside each room and a strobe light and sounder on the outside.

At What Cost?

When the 'Regulations' came into force on the 18th September 1989, it was not possible to fully assimilate what the final cost would be to LUL.

It was agreed with the LFCDA to undertake a pilot programme at five stations where the works would be completed to meet full compliance with the 'Regulations'. These stations are still known as the 'Fully Compliant' stations, and they were chosen to take account of the various types of station environment, i.e.

a)   Stations interfacing with BR (Railtrack)
b)   Stations with escalators
c)   Stations with lifts

and the five stations chosen to cover these aspects were:-

1)   Paddington
2)   London Bridge
3)   Stockwell
4)   Kennington
5)   Goodge Street

In addition to this, a further fifteen stations were identified where the full requirements for 'Compartmentation' were undertaken in accordance with
Regulation 7(1).

As stated earlier, whilst all the above was in progress, LUL were still undertaking interim works.

Regulation 6(3) 'Means For Detecting Fire And Giving Warning In Case Of Fire' also had to be completed in full at 115 stations by 1st January 1991 and, whilst this in itself was a mammoth task, once completed LUL management were able to revert to normal working arrangements and cease the 'Dad's Army' patrols. The interim stand-alone detection systems were also de-commissioned and eventually, to avoid confusion, were removed. However, this had major time and cost implications.

Although these works to install fire detection were completed by 1st January 1991, it still left LUL with a major programme of compartmentation and suppression to be undertaken.

Management sought agreement with the LFCDA to review the project in the light of cost, time and logistics identified in undertaking the work at the five 'fully compliant' stations previously discussed. The LFCDA agreed, with some reservations.

At this point it must be stressed that at the same time other works identified by Fennell were also being undertaken:-

a) Station Public Address   ) both linked to fire alarm
b) Automatic opening ticket barriers   )
c) Preparing revised Station Emergency Plans
d) Preparing and revising Station Fire Plans
e) Staff training
f) Working with Thames Water to provide suitable water supplies in stations for the ESPS.

This last item proved to be more difficult than was first envisaged. The digging of trenches and subsequent road closures had to be carried out predominantly at weekends at the insistence of Local Councils and the Metropolitan Police. Traffic disruption, especially in the West End of London, was a prime consideration. Unfortunately, weekend working upset the residents because of the noise and inconvenience. Most work had to be carried out when premium rates applied.

Management Review

Having completed what was known as 'Section 12 - Phase I' it was obvious to LUL Management that the costs to undertake these works were far higher than had been initially anticipated and that the project could not be completed in the time scales required by the Regulations.

The whole process of Fire Protection was reviewed, to see where savings could be achieved without reducing safety. Without doubt the biggest problem and the most expensive area was achieving adequate compartmentation, which for most of the station environment in order to be in accordance with the 'Regulations, was to a one hour standard. After much deliberation the business accepted proposals that sprinklers were installed throughout the station as a trade off against some of the compartmentation.

Designs were produced based on a format known as the 'Engineered Solution'. These were submitted to the LFCDA and accepted. Obviously this major change in direction to achieve compliance created problems for the Project Management team who had to redesign the work packages, produce new tender specifications and revise the programme.

Appleton Inquiry - QRA

Shortly after the 'Engineered Solution' had been implemented in 1992 the 'Appleton Inquiry' was published.

This was a report produced by Brian Appleton on behalf of the Health and Safety Executive and was an inquiry into "Health and Safety Aspects of Stoppages Caused by Fire and Bomb Alerts on London Underground, British Rail and other Mass Transit Systems".

Within his 'Conclusion and Recommendations' Brian Appleton stated.

"The Section 12 Regulations have led to much sensible improvements. However, now that the risk from fire has been substantially reduced, the outstanding requirements under the Regulations, particularly for extensive fire resistant walls, do not seem wholly justified."

"I recommend that LUL use Quantified Risk Assessment methods to assist it to judge where additional work is not justified and seek exemptions as allowed in the Regulations."

The Engineering Director of LUL immediately instigated meetings with the LFCDA to discuss the merits of moving forward using QRA. The proposal was accepted and a Quantified Risk Assessment of every station was undertaken by external consultants.

Each QRA report took account of the station, its size, passenger flows, numbers of rooms, where they interfaced with other lines or BR and produced a rating using 100 as the base marker. In agreeing with QRA, the LFCDA took note of the rating list and agreed to accept all stations below the top thirteen being designed in an agreed manner to take account of the risk assessment.

LUL now have a 'top thirteen' stations which are fully compliant, and the remaining 99 stations in which the fire safety measures have been designed using the QRA approach.

This created considerable additional work, not only for LUL fire safety managers in agreeing further re-designs with LFCDA, but once again for Project managers in implementing changes to specifications and programmes.

QRA also generated a requirement for LUL and the LFCDA to work very closely together to ensure that approvals were not delayed and to seek ways of reducing the large volumes of paperwork generated by the granting of exemptions required to give legislative approval to the QRA solutions. This was achieved by providing 'Compliance Plans' which have become the legal documents detailing how each station meets compliance. These plans indicate in detail all fire protection arrangements and list 'Exemptions' currently in place and are produced only after full consultation between LUL and LFCDA.

Rolling Stock

It is worth making reference of the advances made in fire safety terms to LUL Rolling Stock. At the time of Kings Cross, not only was the LUL infrastructure old and in need of major refurbishment, but so was their fleet of rolling stock. They contained much combustible material and, although not covered within the new legislation, a Corporate decision was made to replace this material with more modern and much safer alternatives.

Over the last ten years major 'Retrofit' works have been carried out to improve not only the fire performance, but the ambience and comfort for passengers.

This work had to be programmed to allow Rolling Stock management to withdraw sufficient cars for modification, yet still have sufficient stock available to meet the needs of the business. LUL are now moving forward with new rolling stock being introduced into service on the Jubilee Line and Northern Line.

The work undertaken in this area over the past ten years to reduce ignition sources, and introduce new materials which have a better fire performance has been outstanding and a credit to those involved.

Lessons Learned

It is always easy with hindsight to say, "I would not have done it this way". But, without doubt, the route taken in keeping stations open and maintaining a strategic transport network system for the travelling public was correct at the time albeit that it proved very expensive. Over the past four years London Underground have, for construction reasons, closed parts of lines and stations to undertake works. Such closures have allowed other projects to carry out improvements to stations utilising normal working arrangements whereby a contractor actually works full shifts at normal rates, thus not only reducing costs but improving project efficiency.
LUL will continue to take advantage, when parts of lines or stations are closed due to major civil works. But to provide a public transport system for London means "Retrofit" remains the only option open to Management.

Since 1987 London Underground has learnt many lessons in undertaking "Retrofits" on fire safety systems, which is just one link in a continuous chain of safety issues being dealt with.

The Future

London Underground have complied with The Fire Precautions (Sub Surface Railway Stations) Regulation 1989, and have a formal compliance process in place with the LFCDA. They have also produced a joint guidance document on how compliance is achieved.

In 1989 when the 'Regulations' came into force they were necessary. But times have changed. London Underground management have introduced a "Safety Case" system into the business which does not allow changes to take without approval. Within LUL a fire safety team has been established which is dedicated to maintaining fire protection systems and compliance with fire legislation. Unfortunately, the prescriptive nature of the legislation does not allow major change in providing state of the art fire systems, and it is now consider that the time is right to move into the "Self-Compliant" scenario as required by modern legislation including the new "Fire Precautions (Workplace) Regulations 1997". London Underground Ltd. consider that responsible fire safety managers within the business are in a position to negotiate with the LFCDA and HMRI to provide an environment for the travelling public which is both safe and cost effective.

Authors' Index

C537IND